Dr Manorama Legha was
ogist and psychiatrist with
and mood changes. Curre
to the Home Office.

DR M. LEGHA

The Manorama Formula

GRAFTON BOOKS
A Division of the Collins Publishing Group

LONDON GLASGOW
TORONTO SYDNEY AUCKLAND

Grafton Books
A Division of the Collins Publishing Group
8 Grafton Street, London W1X 3LA

A Grafton Paperback Original 1987

ISBN 0-586-07047-8

DISCLAIMER
While the Author and Publishers believe that the principles and
advice contained in this book are soundly based, if you are
receiving medical treatment or have any doubts about your
health or about the suitability of the Manorama Formula for
you, then you should consult your doctor before following the
principles suggested. The Author and Publishers cannot accept
responsibility for injury to health arising out of the observation
by the reader of any of the principles or advice in this book.

Printed and bound in Great Britain by
Collins, Glasgow

Set in Times

Contents

Introduction

This book makes you a promise: that, through a simple principle of natural science, you will lose weight, without dieting, without exercise, without drugs. Moreover, you will lose it permanently.

You will lose as much weight as you wish, whenever you wish.

You will be able to eat whatever you wish, as much as you wish, whenever you wish.

You will not be asked to diet. You will be asked not to diet.

You will not be asked to exercise. You will be asked not to exercise.

And having reached your desired weight, you will be able to maintain it at that level without conscious effort.

You will lose weight because you have so decided. You will have gained permanent weight control.

It has become abundantly clear in recent years that current reducing diets fail in their basic aim of permanent weight reduction. In weight-reducing clinics, for example, where semi-starvation diets are the rule, it is estimated that the yearly return rate of failed dieters is between 90 and 100 per cent.

Whatever their composition, reducing diets are founded on the simplistic calorie expenditure equation, and achieve their object by restricting calories to 1500 a day or less. Some allow as little as 300.

A diet of less than 1500 calories is half that needed to fulfil the essential energy needs of the body. The body is programmed to react to reducing diets as to a threat of incipient starvation. At the earliest onset of dietary restriction, it brings into play adaptive compensatory mechanisms to conserve the diminished supply of energy that is available. The body's basal metabolic rate is slowed down so that less calories are burnt off as energy. This is why so many people complain that they cannot lose weight on moderate calorie restriction and resort to the drastic crash diets so disastrous to health and well-being.

When the desired weight loss has been achieved with one of these diets, and normal eating is resumed, another programmed bodily reaction to starvation brings about a rapid rebound weight gain which proceeds at an accelerated pace until the pounds lost with so much hardship and sacrifice are restored. This again is part of the body's automatic compensatory reaction to starvation. It is why reducing diets invariably fail.

A frequent pattern is that the dieter goes from one diet to another, so that, in physiological terms, periods of fasting are alternated with periods of refeeding. These fluctuations, the so-called 'yo-yo' effect, finally weaken the weight-control mechanism itself, making necessary progressively more stringent diets to achieve the same effect. Additionally they are physiologically harmful, leading eventually to fatigue and deterioration of the regulatory mechanisms for glucose control, with the danger of incipient diabetes. Other systems too must inevitably suffer from these fluctuations.

So reducing diets not only fail, they have a long-term effect on health. Diets fail because they attack the wrong target. The true target in attacking overweight must be the readjustment of the weight regulatory mechanism and the restoration of the sophisticated metabolic processes that exist to keep the body perfectly proportioned, no matter what the quantity and quality of the food that is ingested.

The weight-control mechanism is centred in the brain and operates through nervous circuits between brain and body, with checks, balances and regulatory feed-back signals which normally keep weight at a constant level. Through a complex system of negative feed-back loops, the amount of food ingested is correctly gauged by hypothalamic nerve centres which govern appetite and satiety. It is when this complex mechanism is disturbed that appetite increases and weight gain begins.

Appetite can be normalized by natural means. The appetite-control mechanism will then exactly match food intake to the needs of the body and weight will be perfectly proportioned to height, build and individual make-up. It will be permanently maintained at this level automatically. Weight can then be predictably and naturally lost by making use of the body's own mechanism for accelerating energy combustion to burn up excess pounds.

I formulated the Manorama Formula 15 years ago. I based it on a philosophical deduction that ideal body weight is the norm and is maintained naturally throughout life. In the event of a disturbance, a scientifically valid approach would be the only way to normalize it. I examined the weight-regulating mechanism and the numerous energy circuits subscribing to it, the nervous messages they transmitted, and the biological changes they produced. I took into account all the other vital systems and their interaction with the weight-control mechanism. I put it into practice and, as predicted, achieved 100 per cent success with all who learnt the system. Subsequent scientific discoveries in the field of food metabolism and energy balance have, as expected, validated it entirely.

As a demonstration of how weight can be normalized by natural means, I will explain two recently discovered physiological phenomena which have so far not been exploited either by medical experts or by the weight-reduction industry. The action of the 'brown fat' in accelerating the rate of calorie combustion is one of these. Brown fat, small quantities of special fat which are scattered throughout the body, burns up calories at a rate significantly above normal, acting like a furnace in the body. It is activated in certain circumstances. In conditions of severe cold, for instance, it produces the 'thermogenic effect', rapidly burning calories to produce extra heat for the sake of raising the body temperature to normal. But more importantly, it is involved in food ingestion, so that when certain rules are followed, the same thermogenic effect can be induced to burn off extra calories. These are dissipated, causing a net weight loss. So that when these rules are followed, eating can actually reduce weight.

In all reducing diets, the brown fat is inactivated as part of the adaptive mechanisms of the body for conserving the diminished supply of energy to fuel its vital needs. So calorie restriction converts the dieters into slow burners, with the result that though they eat little they remain overweight. Many diet clinics not only fail to recognize the problem, they compound it by giving thyroid to raise the basal metabolic rate. This is counterproductive; added thyroid in fact completely inactivates the brown fat, again as an adaptive measure the body uses to conserve energy.

When the brown fat remains inactivated for any length of time, as in calorie restriction or thyroid administration, it becomes atrophied from disuse. This is the major reason why, in spite of determined efforts, constant dieters remain fat. The Manorama Formula will show you not only how to reactivate, but how to regenerate the brown fat and convert yourself into a fast burner. You will be able to eat whatever you wish and as much as you wish and lose weight automatically.

The second phenomenon is the action of the 'endogenous opiates', so called because they are natural substances in the body whose action and composition are not only similar to, but a hundred times more potent than, morphine. The opiates are distributed throughout gut and brain and are the physiological substrates of the satisfaction in eating that is part of the instinct of survival.

The endogenous opiates are a powerful part of the mechanism by which the body keeps weight at an ideal level, in harmony with height and build. When these opiates are not activated, or are insufficiently activated, overeating takes place. Additionally, the setting of the appetite centre in the brain which governs appetite and satiety is raised to a higher level, resulting in a constant intake of food in excess of the body's needs. You will be shown how the process can be reversed by reactivating the opiates. You will be shown how to make use of the opiate system's role in the mechanism which exists to keep the body perfectly proportioned, no matter what the quantity and quality of the food that is ingested.

You will be taken step by step through the bodily mechanisms concerned with weight control. The various nervous circuits involved will be explained to you simply and concisely. These systems are normally not under voluntary control. They are governed by the autonomic or involuntary nervous system, and thus are not directly linked with the voluntary nervous system. As such, therefore, they cannot be switched on at will. You will, however, be shown a method by which they can be brought under the direct control of the will. By interposing a trigger between the voluntary act of eating and these circuits, you will be able, every time you eat, to switch on the brown fat and the endogenous opiate circuits. This will have the dual effect of reducing weight by increasing the rate of the body's combustion of calories, at the same time regulating the weight control apparatus.

When you have consciously activated these systems a number of times, the experience will become recorded in the brain. The brain will become programmed in the process. From then on it will automatically switch on these systems on cue every time you eat, regardless of what you eat and how much. You will begin to lose weight without further conscious effort.

The Manorama Formula is precise and powerful in execution, and predictable in its outcome. With it you will be able to regulate your weight effortlessly, pleasantly and naturally. You will be free from restraints, restrictions and limitations. You will be in control.

1

Calorie control – the obsolete formula

Weight control by dieting is no control. It is subordination to dieting. Dieting controls what you eat, how much you eat, when you eat. And as soon as you stop dieting, you start to regain the lost weight, promptly, rapidly and relentlessly, till you are back where you started from.

This is the in-built, inherent defect of reducing diets. Right at the outset they initiate a series of physiological changes. No matter how prolonged the diet, as soon as it is stopped, those changes will swing the weight pendulum back to its original starting point. Inevitably and inexorably. This is a rebound reaction; if the weight loss is caused by dieting, it must be regained.

Statistics show that 90 per cent of dieters revert back to their original weight. Two per cent stop marginally short. Eight per cent overshoot that weight.

All current reducing diets operate by restricting calories and by calorie restriction alone. They have no other reducing factor.

They may claim that certain foods have fat-burning properties or that some food has specific reducing capabilities. But this is mere window-dressing to disguise the underlying calorie restriction. You can gain weight on a high-protein/high-fibre low-salt diet, and you can lose weight on a high-fat/high-sugar/high-salt diet. The operative factor is its calorie value.

The fact is that in terms of weight loss or weight gain, 100 calories of fat are exactly equal to 100 calories of salad.

All reducing diets restrict calories, some overtly, others

covertly. Covert calorie control is brought about by controlling the choice of food. By allowing only certain types of food, a relative surfeit of the nutrients in question is created. Covert calorie control diets rely on an in-built bodily mechanism by which an excess of any nutrient is detected by the assessors in the gut and signals to this effect are sent to the taste-buds. The same food in the same meal which was only recently palatable now becomes unpalatable. Further eating is inhibited. If in spite of these negative signals the dieter persists with the same food, definite feelings of nausea are aroused. These undesirable consequences can cause long-term aversion to that particular food or combination of foods, resulting in further reduction in calorie intake.

As for the alleged specific dynamic action of protein, which is the basis of claims for the reducing properties of high-protein diets, this has no scientific foundation. The theory claims that 20–30 per cent of the calories contained in protein are used up in such a way that they do not convert to bodily fat. If this were true, the effect would be the same as if you had eaten a third to a fifth less than in fact you actually ate. This ill-founded theory has been tested and long since disproved. There is no statistically significant difference between the amount of calories expended by protein metabolism and that of other foods.

It is a medical fact that there is no food which is reducing as such.

There is no combination of foods which is reducing as such.

Low-fat diets, no-fat diets, protein diets, high-protein diets, vegetable and nut diets, meat and salad diets, low-salt diets, high-fibre diets, fruit-only diets, milk and fruit diets, milk-only diets, formula diets, all variously promoted as having some special reducing property, have one single common operative factor – calorie restriction.

It had long become evident to me that the calorie input/ calorie output equation was grossly simplistic. It naïvely presumes that food restriction will automatically result in a corresponding degree of weight reduction. I knew this could not happen. There is a far more complex arrangement in the body's handling of food intake, and a far more sophisticated system of energy balance than the calorie input/output formula presupposes. I had long considered the old calorie-control system of weight reduction obsolete. It simply did not fit the biological facts. All subsequent scientific discoveries in the field of energy balance have amply confirmed my original deductions and have supported the Manorama Formula I devised 15 years ago.

All current diets allow less than 1500 calories. This is about half the normal requirements of the body. For the proper functioning of the vital systems alone, the body needs 1500 calories a day. In addition, further calories are required for external movement, depending on the amount of physical activity engaged in – a minimum of 1300 for a sedentary worker of small build, proportionately more for a manual labourer – making a total daily minimal requirement of 3,000 calories.

Most reducing diets allow only 1000 calories – a third of the normal requirement – some as little as 300. A diet of less than 1500 calories does not even meet the daily requirements of the vital functions. This is physiological starvation.

By definition, all reducing diets are starvation diets.

Starvation is against the natural law of self-preservation. The body reacts to starvation as to a threat to survival itself. It has two programmed responses to starvation. These come into force automatically.

The first programme becomes operational at the onset of starvation and remains effective as long as it lasts. The second takes over as soon as starvation ceases and remains in force until the lost weight is regained.

Starvation diets cause the blood sugar level to drop to an abnormally low level. This adversely affects the body at all levels, inducing physical lethargy and exhaustion, emotional depression, anxiety and intellectual clouding. These effects are incompatible with health. To minimize their consequences, the body tries to conserve energy and bridge the calorie gap. It does this by bringing into play the central mechanism which lowers the basal metabolic rate. Less calories are burnt, less energy is expended, and all bodily systems slow down proportionately. The dieter slows down to such an extent that often, in spite of drastic food restriction, no significant weight loss occurs.

When there *is* weight loss, it is not only lost at great cost, it is lost only temporarily. As soon as the diet is discontinued, the second programmed bodily reaction takes over and a rapid rebound weight gain ensues. The second programme is concerned with the actual body weight at the time when dieting was started. When normal eating is resumed the blood sugar level is restored to normal but the body is programmed to maintain the basal metabolic rate at a low level until the lost weight is regained.

The body cannot discriminate between weight loss caused by enforced starvation and that lost by deliberate starvation. Its reaction to both is identical.

It is in keeping with the natural law of restoration that weight lost by starvation must be rapidly regained.

This sequence of events is invariable and predictable.

The cost of a starvation diet is exhaustion, depression and mental clouding while the diet is in progress, anxiety, loss of control and feelings of helplessness during the phase of weight regain, and feelings of failure and hopelessness when it has been regained. These costs in terms of health and well-being alone make dieting unacceptable.

All existing reducing diets cause weight loss by starvation and starvation alone.

Whether it is a one-page diet sheet or a 200-page diet book, whether undertaken at a diet clinic or health farm, all current diet plans can be summarized in two lines:

'This diet has less than 1500 calories. It will cause weight loss by starvation. There is no other operative factor.'

One further line would conclude the subject: 'It must fail.'

You did not fail. The diet failed you.

Weight loss by exercise is also based on calorie input/calorie output manipulation, in this case the weight loss being achieved by increasing calorie expenditure through output.

The body reacts to calorie deficit caused by exercise in the same way as it does to calorie deficit caused by input control. As soon as it is discontinued, the weight loss will be regained.

As with dieting, the body does not discriminate between weight lost by enforced exertion and that lost by deliberate exertion. Its response is the same. The lost pounds are speedily replaced as soon as the exercise is discontinued. So exercise as a means of weight control has the same in-built defect as dieting.

This too is in keeping with the natural law of restoration. Weight lost by extra exertion must be regained.

Reducing diets are fundamentally misdirected. They attack the wrong target – hunger. Hunger is essential for survival. By attacking it, reducing diets attack the foundations of survival.

Overeating is not caused by increased hunger. In health, hunger exactly matches the body's energy needs. It decodes these needs with precision, and automatically adjusts to them as they fluctuate during the course of the day. When these fluctuating needs are met, hunger disappears. So hunger can cause neither weight gain nor weight loss. By making hunger their target, reducing diets de-stabilize its reading apparatus. To be finely tuned to the changing energy needs of the body, hunger needs to be nurtured.

Reducing diets also attack appetite. Though both are linked to the basic instinct of survival, the instinct to nourish, appetite is not identical to hunger. Appetite not only serves the energy needs of the body, it decodes its other nutritional needs as well. It decodes the changes in these needs. When the body is hot, it demands cooling food and drink. When it is dehydrated, it demands extra water and salt. When it is becoming depleted of energy, it demands ready energy sources such as carbohydrates and sugary foods. To be sharply tuned, the appetite too needs to be nurtured.

Reducing diets dictate non-preferred foods in non-preferred quantities at non-preferred times. They de-stabilize the appetite and blunt its finer tuning. So the body's needs are not met and the appetite circle is kept open.

There is a biological basis for this. When there is a shortfall of essential nutrients, no matter how small the required quantity, there will be a compulsion to eat until that shortfall is made good.

The true target of any weight-control regime should be the weight-control mechanism of the body, a special regulatory centre in the brain which determines and maintains your ideal body weight in proportion to your height, build and unique, individual make-up. This perfect control of weight is a constant, persistent and universal feature throughout the animal kingdom. It is fully developed at birth. Most people maintain it throughout life. Its precision is emphasized by the recent estimation that the average woman gains only 11 kg between the ages of 25 and 65, during which time she will have eaten 20 tons of food, a weight change corresponding to an average daily error of the infinitesimal amount of only 350 mg of food, a remarkable demonstration of the mathematical precision of the weight-control mechanism.

The weight-control centre in the brain maintains perfect balance between food intake and energy expenditure. It does this by the interplay of highly sensitive and sophisticated systems of nervous circuits, checks, balances and feedback mechanisms. The weight-control mechanism regulates hunger to match exactly bodily needs. It precisely matches appetite to hunger.

This sensitively organized mechanism can be temporarily disturbed by internal stress or by environmental factors. If normal eating is continued, it will usually correct itself once the stress is removed. If, on the other hand, dieting is resorted to, an abnormal factor is introduced. The mechanism can then be permanently disrupted.

When the weight-control mechanism is dislocated, the appetite is raised in excess of bodily needs and the setting of the appetite regulatory centre rises proportionately in compensation. When dieting is stopped, the dislocated weight-control mechanism and the higher setting remain uncorrected. The mechanism is then permanently disrupted. Food is ingested in excess of the body's needs. The result is weight gain.

Chronic dieting compounds the higher setting of the appetite regulatory centre. The calorie shortfall lowers the blood sugar. To raise it to normal, the setting is adjusted further upwards, setting in motion an upward-bound spiral. When the diet is discontinued, the setting remains raised. Further excessive eating to meet the increased demand is inevitable and the lost weight returns. A vicious circle is set in motion which is self-perpetuating. The pattern of weight loss/rebound weight gain has become established. The scene is set for a lifetime battle with weight gain.

The Manorama Formula can correct the dysfunction of your appetite-control mechanism. It will be explained to you, explicitly and concisely, how the appetite setting can be lowered and the spiral reversed. A reduction to 10 per cent below normal can be achieved and can be absorbed by the system without provoking the body's adaptive measures. This factor alone can cause considerable and continuous weight loss without any rebound reaction or disturbance of inner stability.

The Manorama Formula will show you how the central control mechanism can be rejuvenated and restabilized to correct the fundamental metabolic dysfunction which has caused your weight gain. It will show you how you can do this naturally and effortlessly without diet or exercise.

By applying the Manorama Formula you will be able to restore the finer tuning of your appetite in line with your bodily needs. You will be able to eat what you like, as much as you like, yet you will lose weight. You will have unrestricted choice.

Restrictions on foods such as cholesterol, sugar and salt on health grounds are equally invalid. They are based on outmoded and unscientific theories. Only in the case of certain constitutional diseases such as diabetes, familial hypercholesterolaemia, or salt-sensitive hypertension, which affect a minute fraction of the population, are there any clinical grounds for restricting their intake. In diabetes, for example, there is a case for restricting sugar as the mechanism for regulating blood-sugar levels is defective. The same applies to familial hypercholesterolaemia, a genetic condition in which the metabolism of cholesterol is impaired and high blood levels of this fat are present. In the healthy individual, blood levels of cholesterol are maintained at a constant low level no matter what the content of the food eaten.

Cholesterol is not an alien toxin. It is a vital constituent of the body that must be constantly replenished. The greatest natural nutritional experiment in the world's history has been on a substance which is loaded with cholesterol, milk. Infants have thrived on it since the world began. The food theorists would have us believe that it suddenly becomes toxic after infancy. You will not be asked to give up milk, eggs, butter, or other cholesterol-rich foods.

Salt too is a vital constituent of the body, also needing constant replenishment. It does not raise the blood pressure. This theory has been scientifically discredited. The healthy body possesses its own highly efficient mechanism for eliminating any excess. You will not be asked to restrict salt.

Sugar is a valuable ready source of energy and contains nothing inherently harmful. You will not have to give up sugar.

All food which fulfils the body's needs is good food. The only bad food is that which is decomposed or adulterated. By treating sugar, salt and fats as noxious foreign substances, ill-thought-out food theories are creating unnecessary fears and phobias about good, valuable food.

Conversely the non-food bran is extolled. There is no known human enzyme capable of digesting bran. Hence it is not a food. Bran is the tough outer husk of the grain whose natural function is to protect the essential nutrients within. 'Bran enriched' foods act as irritants to the gut and produce noxious gases. In some cases, gut obstruction requiring emergency intervention has been reported. Eating bran does not cause weight loss. You will not be asked to eat bran.

The purpose of food is to supply energy and to replenish the wear and tear of the bodily tissues. Fats, proteins and carbohydrates all convert to energy at a different rate. To maintain a stable energy supply in between meals, each one of them has its own unique role to play. In addition, fats, proteins and carbohydrates have further non-interchangeable roles to play in the bodily economy. They can none of them be dispensed with. None of them will make you fat.

You will not be asked to give up wines or spirits. As in the case of other foods (and inedible substances) they can produce an allergic response in a fraction of the population which can be readily identified by the hypersensitive or obviously adverse reaction they produce. Personally incompatible spirits, wines, or groups of wines can be ignored; the rest are good food.

Wines and spirits have a quality which no other food has. Being alcohol-based, they are absorbed into the bloodstream more quickly than any other food and thus quickly make good any physical or emotional energy deficit. The quantity of spirit producing the optimum benefit is an individual variable; beyond the stage of usefulness it naturally produces the inhibiting reaction of surfeit and desire for spirit ceases.

During periods of stress the body indicates its greater need for the kind of quick restorative action that alcohol can provide in terms of elevating physical and emotional depression. When the stress factor is removed, the body indicates its lowered needs.

A fraction of the population are so constituted that their emotional quality of life continues to improve with alcohol and they make use of it beyond the surfeit stage. When their quality of life is otherwise enriched, their need for spirit adjusts to normal.

Wines and spirits have stood the test of time as excellent

restoratives. Unless taken without food or in combination with incompatible drugs they fulfil their function efficiently and effectively. To attribute to them directly the damage caused by their excessive use in individuals whose quality of life is otherwise diminished is not clinically defensible.

When you have grasped the essentials of the Manorama principles you will not need to restrict your food intake in any way. You will not need artificially to increase your calorie output by exercise. You will lose weight by revitalizing your metabolic processes and by correcting the dysfunction in the central weight regulatory mechanism. You will be doing this by recruiting your own natural resources and not by going against nature.

·2
Existing diet regimes

You have made a decision to lose weight and you will do so. All you need is the decision and the correct information.

If you have failed to lose weight in the past by dieting, that was inevitable. Diets confront, conflict with, and are contrary to the instinct of survival. In normal health the instinct will always prevail.

Most people in normal health have built-in weight control. You too will achieve this. What is humanly possible is possible for all humans.

You possess in your brain a mechanism whose sole purpose is to control your body weight. It does so by regulating energy intake and energy expenditure. It computes the results of the energy-related processes and works out the energy generation/expenditure ratio. After having computed the numerous variables entailed, it makes constant adjustments to the energy-static mechanisms, finally adjusting the energy-static setting to conform with your ideal body weight.

This mechanism you already possess. All that it is necessary for you to do is to strengthen it. You can do this once you are in possession of the correct information. When you have absorbed and stored the correct information, you will acquire the correct mental posture. You will automatically initiate action in the furtherance of your decision.

To make full use of the correct information all you have to do is to free yourself of the influences of all previous misconceptions about weight reduction. This negative information conflicts with the positive and acts as an obstacle to its assimilation, proportionately reducing its impact.

Reducing diets must be actively discarded. They are negative in every aspect and in every detail. They are an obstacle to implementing your decision to lose weight. When their adverse effects are fully explained to you, you will automatically reject them.

While you are discarding the obsolete dogmas of weight reduction, you will be actively absorbing the correct information. This will have a positive effect on your weight-control mechanism, which will automatically start to assert itself and will begin to serve your decision to lose weight.

Diets and dieting are the obsolete dogmas of weight reduction.

Diets are ill-conceived, ill-construed and ill-constructed.

They are *ill-conceived* because the concept of weight loss by dieting can in itself lead to weight gain. From the instant you conceive the idea of eating less, you set in motion the mechanism whereby you actually eat more. If you decide to eat less next day you will overeat today, if at the next meal you will overeat at this meal. This is inevitable because it is linked with the instinct to preserve. Animals in nature who anticipate lack of food in winter overeat and slow down to put on weight and store energy. This is an instinctive and invariable occurrence.

The instant you conceive the idea of eating less you set yourself up to gain weight. You overeat and you slow down. Anticipation of dieting will keep this mechanism alive.

Not only does dieting cause anticipatory overeating, it

causes retrospective overeating when the diet is discontinued. This is maintained until the enforced weight loss is made good. The experience of starvation brings into play a mechanism whereby weight is gained over and above that lost by dieting as an insurance against further periods of starvation. The pattern is universal because it is biological.

Concomitant with this biological pattern is an equally universal emotional one:

Anxiety and overeating before dieting.

Tension and starvation during dieting.

Guilt and overeating after dieting.

Diets are *ill-construed* in their basic implications. It is invariably stipulated by their authors that they should be carried out under medical supervision, thereby introducing the implication that overweight people are ill. This has an inevitable demoralizing effect on the dieter. It is also an indictment of the diets themselves, underlining the fact that they are unnatural, risky and unhealthy.

Reducing diets are *ill-constructed* because they disregard the internal clock.

The internal clock is the central mechanism which signals the individual needs of the body. Individual needs have a wide variation. People who rise early and are more active in the early part of the day vary in their food requirements from those who sleep later and are more active in the afternoon and evening. The former will require more food in the mornings than the latter. Diets demand fixed amounts of food at set times regardless of the internal clock. This disturbs the energy balance and is non-conducive to weight loss.

Disregarding the internal clock can be harmful. Reviews of cases of gastric ulcer have shown that those fed by the clock in infancy developed ulcers significantly more frequently than those fed on demand.

Dieting is damaging, destructive and disintegrating

It is *damaging* because repeated failures entrench the underlying cause of your overeating and make it more difficult to overcome. Initially, overeating is usually compensatory and temporary, a safety valve in times of emotional or environmental stress. Of all the compensatory measures, it is the healthiest, most socially acceptable, and the most easily remediable. The stress of dieting and the stress of dietary failure compound the initial stress which, probably transient to begin with, now becomes entrenched.

Dieting is *destructive*. The abnormal fluctuations arising from the rapid changes inflicted by starvation and return to normal eating act as a trauma to the central regulatory mechanisms, including the master weight-control mechanism in the brain, resulting in its weakening and destabilization.

Dieting is *disintegrating*. It physically disintegrates self-perception. This is demonstrated by the common distortion of the body image found in dieters, whereby the dieter invariably imagines herself to be fatter than she really is. Experiments have been performed with distorting mirrors which reflect the same person in varying sizes. Invited to select the reflection most approximate to their actual size, the dieters invariably selected those significantly larger than they actually were. They related the image so perceived to unsightliness. The extreme example of the distortion of the body image caused by dieting is in anorexia nervosa, where pathological underweights imagine themselves to be gross overweights and correspondingly ugly because of their imagined size.

Reducing diets are painful, punitive and perilous

Diets are *painful*. They both generate and misuse pain. Pain is a life-saving warning signal whose purpose is to

warn against damage to health. Pain invites removal of
the causative agent. It persists, demanding attention as a
priority, until the damaging agent is removed or neutralized. If there were no pain, life itself would be at risk.

The pain of semi-starvation is both physical and
emotional, the pain of the starvation itself and the pain
of despair at the eventual return of the lost weight. The
chemical changes induced by continuous pain disturb
stability of mind and mood.

Reducing diets are perhaps the only regimes which do
not conform to the usual requirement of alleviation of
pain by dispersal or disposal of the causative agent, but
actively and essentially demand the creation, promotion
and propagation of pain in perpetuity.

Dieting is *punitive*, not only because diets are painful
in themselves, but because they isolate their victim. Diets
take over one's social life. They make impossible normal
communal and family eating. They not only inflict pain,
they make it impossible to share the pain and pain
unshared is doubly punitive.

Diets are *perilous*. Most are severely deficient in vitamins and essential minerals. The deficiency is further
compounded by a reduction of the synthesis and absorption of vitamins and minerals in the body, exacerbating
the loss of vitality and virility inherent in dieting, in some
cases so severely as to lead to infertility.

Diets of 1000 calories or less can cause loss of hair and
skin elasticity. They significantly decrease resistance to
infection. Serious emotional changes, depression, anxiety
and pessimism may occur. Some diets are directly responsible for generating toxic end products like ketones and
phytic acid, which cause chronic ill health. The most
important hazard of these diets, however, is depletion of
muscle tissue. When this occurs in the heart muscle, the
results can be serious and even fatal. All these hazards

are exemplified in the most popular diets currently in use.

A series of diet books in the last decade have all been announced as 'miracle diets' or 'wonder diets'. All claim to shed large amounts of weight in short periods of time. All claim that those who have used the diets have 'felt wonderful' throughout, an implication of improved health not tenable on physiological grounds and one belied by the doctors writing in the medical journals who have had to deal with the disastrous effects of these diets.

Yet all these diets have in-built recipes for failure. Though they prescribe varying amounts of food or combinations of food, or give prominence to one particular food at the expense of others, they all operate by calorie restriction. In other words, they are prescriptions for starvation. They are also prescriptions for chronic overweight problems, as the body will react to replace the lost pounds with a rapidity commensurate with the pace at which they were shed.

Though some diets claim to eschew calorie counting, the limitations imposed on certain foods lead to in-built calorie restriction. They are covert calorie-counting diets, achieving their aim by the surfeit and monotony of the foods allowed.

All these aspects are illustrated by the currently popular 'big five' 'miracle diets'. All claim to possess some unique formula or ingredient for weight loss that makes them entirely novel and revolutionary, a claim reiterated with such confidence as to induce credibility. In fact, there is nothing either miraculous or novel about any of them. All depend on drastic calorie restriction either overt or concealed. They work entirely by physiological starvation, with all its inevitable consequences.

The Scarsdale diet, the first of the five, appeared in 1978. It is a 1,000-calorie diet, and it is claimed that it can lose 20 lb in weight in two weeks. It is, in fact, the latest in a long line of high-protein, low-carbohydrate diets, all based on a scientific fallacy, that of the alleged 'specific dynamic action' of protein. In fact, the co-author with Dr Tarnowers of *The Complete Scarsdale Medical Diet* is Sam Sinclair Baker, who also co-authored the first of the books based on this discredited theory, Dr Stillman's *The Doctor's Quick Weight Loss Diet*, published in 1968.

Stillman took the concept of the specific dynamic energy of protein from Eugene Dubois, MD, who maintained that, as the protein molecule is so big and complex, the body must use extra energy to digest it. He estimated that 20–30 per cent of the calories in protein would be expended in its metabolization. This theory was shown to be untrue in 1973, when Drs R. S. Bradfield and Martin H. Jourdan, nutritionalists at the University of California, performed experiments to discover whether there was any such thing as a specific dynamic action of protein. Their tests, published in the medical journal *Lancet*, showed negative results, findings never challenged since.

The weight loss achieved by the Scarsdale diet is claimed to be based solely on the twin pillars of the alleged specific dynamic energy of protein and on the diet's ketogenic effects. In fact, neither factor plays any role; the only operative factor is the semi-starvation induced by the 1000-calorie intake allowed.

The Scarsdale diet is nutritionally unbalanced, not only being deficient in energy, but specifically in vitamins A and D. The fact that the authors recommend two weeks on the diet and two weeks off exacerbates the stresses of the 'yo-yo' phenomenon, with more fatiguing of the homeostatic control mechanisms.

But the most serious consequence of the diet, and what makes it more dangerous than other drastic diets, is that it is, as the authors frankly admit, a ketogenic diet.

Ketone bodies are toxic end products of faulty metabolism, generated when insufficient carbohydrate is consumed to burn fat effectively. An identical condition is a complication of diabetes, in which it is always regarded as serious.

Ketone bodies circulating in the bloodstream adversely affect the whole body, but brain cells, being the body's most sensitive, are the worst affected. Ketones excreted in the urine damage the kidneys. They can cause dangerous cardiac irregularities. In pregnancy, a ketone diet can cause abnormalities in the fetus. Ketosis leads to metabolic acidosis, an alteration in the acid base reaction of the blood, and can provoke a rise in the level of uric acid in the blood, which causes gout. Common symptoms in even mild ketosis are nausea, light-headedness, exhaustion and depression. The excretion of ketones in the breath produces mouth odour and bad breath.

Tarnowers and Baker, however, make a virtue out of this serious risk factor, claiming that 'metabolism and ketones play a major role' in their diet. 'If you are producing ketones,' they state, 'it is a sign that your body is burning off fat at an accelerated rate; you are enjoying *Fast Food Metabolism*. And that is what we want.' They further extol ketosis because it curbs the appetite. When appetite is reduced it is entirely due to the serious abnormal chemical changes induced. Only a severe degree of ketosis will succeed in lowering the appetite.

A similar high-protein, low-carbohydrate diet, *Dr Atkins Diet Revolution*, published in 1972, had also frankly stated that 'ketosis is a state devoutly to be desired'. Atkins even advised his readers to buy urine-testing sticks, or tablets from the chemist that turn purple in the presence of ketone bodies, just to make certain that they were in ketosis. 'Keep the sticks turning purple', he advised, 'and you keep losing weight.' Actually to promote the toxic state of ketogenesis as a condition to be desired is very unusual medical advice indeed.

Rival to the Scarsdale diet is the Pritikin diet, which appeared in 1979. An engineer working in the electronics field, Nathan Pritikin became founder and director of the Longevity Research Institute in Santa Barbara, California. His first book, *The Pritikin Program,* was originally designed not to reduce weight, but allegedly to promote long life through a specific dietary regime. The same diet was later presented as the *Maximum Weight Loss Diet,* based on the same principles.

The Pritikin diet is essentially a vegetarian diet – animal products like fish and meat are recommended to be used as condiments rather than as major constituents of the regime. The diet is a covert calorie restriction regime in that it does not count calories. The dieter is allowed to eat as much as desired of raw vegetables, and indeed is advised to carry round a plastic bag of these foods which can be eaten all day long to stave off the pangs of hunger. But only one portion a day is allowed from the grain, dairy and fruit groups of foodstuffs. Thus, as raw vegetables have a low calorie value in any case, calorie restriction is built in to the diet by the limitations imposed on the other foods.

A more drastic version of the Pritikin diet eschews grain products altogether, and most of its protein is therefore derived from plant sources and is lacking in some of the essential amino acids. Fats are completely avoided, even the polyunsaturated ones. As the fat-soluble vitamins such as A and D cannot be utilized in the body without dietary fat, severe deficiencies in these vitamins can result.

Tea, coffee and alcohol are forbidden, as well as sugar or artificial sweeteners. Little salt is allowed. It is thus an extremely insipid, spartan diet. One wonders if the boredom of living on such a diet is compensated by the alleged longevity achieved. Pritikin himself committed suicide in February 1985.

The Beverly Hills Diet was announced in a blaze of publicity with the publication in 1981 of the book of the same name by Ms Judy Mazell, described as an aspiring actress and record company secretary. As Drs Merkin and Shore pointed out in the *Journal of the American Medical Association* (13 November 1981), she is 'neither a physician nor a nutritionalist, and this soon becomes evident from her book'. 'Her college training,' they say, 'was primarily in dramatics.'

Certainly the author's idea of the digestive processes of the body is bizarre in the extreme, and the diet was described in the same journal as 'nutritional nonsense' and 'the latest and perhaps the worst entry in the diet-fad derby'.

The Beverly Hills diet is based on what the author calls the 'life-altering' principle of 'conscious combining', by which she means 'consciously eating foods together that digest together best'. Proteins and carbohydrates 'fight one another, digestively speaking', the book proclaims, so they should not be eaten together. 'A slower-digesting food will block the digestion of a faster-digesting food if they are eaten together.' For example, 'the spaghetti in spaghetti and meat balls clumps up in your stomach while it waits for the meatballs to digest', and 'potatoes get locked in your stomach and ferment to vodka'. Equally bizarre claims are made for the digestive enzymes, i.e. that the enzymes that digest protein fight with those that digest carbohydrates, setting up a chemical reaction that neutralizes the carbohydrate enzymes. Thus, 'It is not what we eat or how much we eat but what we eat together that counts . . . as long as food is fully digested, fully processed through the body, you will not gain weight. It's only undigested food, food that is "stuck" in your body, for whatever reason, that accumulates and becomes fat.'

These absurd statements are, of course, totally untrue. There is in nature almost no food, apart perhaps from pure granulated sugar, which does not contain carbohydrates, fats and proteins in varying amounts. Therefore the enzymes which break down these foods before they can be absorbed must be and are able to 'work together'.

The statement that only undigested food causes fatness is equally absurd. Undigested food cannot be absorbed from the intestinal tract and it passes out of the body. It is therefore not undigested food but fully digested food that causes fatness.

Foods which allegedly do not digest together are called 'miscombinations'. But they need not be avoided altogether, the author says. 'Obviously many miscombinations are far too splendid for us to continually and/or forever pass them by. I, for one, am not willing to give up pizza or my sandwiches or my soufflés.' The answer is, according to her, to 'use the enzymatic power of fruits to counteract the effects of a particular miscombined overdose.'

Mazell then goes on to refer to the 'fat-burning enzymes' in specified fruits. She refers to the 'power of pineapple' and the 'wonder of papaya'. This also is physiological nonsense. There are no 'fat-burning enzymes' in fruit. Enzymes in fruit and other sources outside the body are proteins, and as such are broken down in the stomach before they ever reach the fatty tissues. But the first phase of the Beverly Hills Diet prescribes 10 days of eating fruit alone in ordered amounts 'designed to burn up fat, soften surplus flesh and then wash out the residue' – which is arrant nonsense. Any weight loss arising from a fruit-only diet arises from the fact that the surfeit of fruit makes it a covert calorie-control diet. Additionally, weight loss may be caused by the diarrhoea produced by such a diet.

A diet consisting entirely of fruit can cause severe diarrhoea and loss of important minerals such as potassium and calcium from the body. If the diet is persisted with after the onset of diarrhoea, dehydration can result in drying of the skin, a rapid, thready pulse, weakness and dizziness, and a drop in blood pressure. Such low blood pressures have been reported as to be almost incompatible with life, though fortunately no deaths have as yet been reported on the diet. The Beverly Hills Diet is severely deficient in protein and there have been many complaints of hair loss, depletion of skin protein, and muscle weakness. Gastrointestinal complaints include ulcers, gassiness and bloating.

The book proclaims its physiological naïveté by making a virtue of the calcium depletion caused by the diet, saying that this lessens the risk of calcium stones in the kidneys. In fact, kidney stones are caused by calcium metabolism. In normal health the ingestion of calcium-containing food can never cause stone formation.

According to the preface to Mazell's second book, the Beverly Hills Diet is reminiscent of the old Chinese yin and yang philosophy, which arbitrarily pronounces certain foods 'yin' and others 'yang', soft, humid foods being yin, and cold and hard ones yang. According to the doctrine, the two different foods should not be eaten together. The philosophy recently became fashionable in the cultish Zen Macrobiotic Diet, which is severely deficient in essential nutrients and has been responsible for causing scurvy, low blood protein, low blood calcium and, through fluid restriction, kidney disease. The American Medical Association has issued several warnings to the public about the dangers of this diet, which has already caused several deaths.

With all its manifest dangers, *The Beverly Hills Diet*

sold in millions, causing a wide dissemination of health problems. But Mazell persisted in her claims in a follow-up book dedicated to her readers in which she declared, 'YOU BOUGHT IT, YOU BELIEVED IT, YOU TRIED IT, YOU MADE IT WORK FOR YOU. And with the fuel of your lost pounds and contagious energy, the Beverley Hills Diet ignited and word rocketed around the world.'

Though it is specified that there is no calorie counting and no portion control, calorie restriction is in-built in the Beverly Hills Diet. It is a covert calorie-control diet, achieving its aim through the sheer monotony and surfeit of eating only one type of food at a meal. This factor is the basis of all the one-food 'crash diets', such as the banana-only diet or the milk-only diet once popular. The physiological basis of the Beverly Hills Diet is as sound as that of the cider vinegar diet claimed to 'dissolve' the fat in the tissues. Yet with all their absurdities, these diets gain a huge following, resulting in commensurately large health problems.

The F-Plan was a spin-off from the fibre cult that had been growing since the late sixties when Dr Denis Burkitt advanced the theory that lack of dietary fibre was responsible for many gastrointestinal diseases, including cancer of the colon. This theory was scientifically unsubstantiated, as will be discussed in the next chapter. But it caught the popular imagination and resulted in a cult that blamed 'all the diseases of western civilization' on lack of fibre in the diet. Since then, not only vegetable and fruit fibre, which formed the basis of Burkitt's theory, but bran, as the crudest and toughest fibre of all, has gained immense popularity. Not surprisingly, lack of fibre in the diet has been indicted as a cause of obesity and Audrey Eyton's book caught the rising tide of this interest at the optimal moment. As a result of *The F-Plan*'s success, bran products have proliferated on the supermarket shelves and large fortunes have been made by their manufacturers.

Audrey Eyton's diet plan claims to double the intake of dietary fibre largely by the addition of bran. Her menus make abundant use of bran – bran breads, bran cereals and bran biscuits, and contain 35–50 grammes of dietary fibre. The mainstay of the diet is a 'fibre-filler muesli' made of bran flakes, bran, All Bran or Bran Buds, with prunes, dried apricots and sultanas.

The claims of the health-giving properties of bran will be discussed in a later chapter. Here I will only deal with its alleged weight-reducing properties.

The slimming properties of bran are said to lie in the feeling of bulk it produces in the stomach, giving an impression of fullness and satiety. Fullness of the stomach is an important part of the appetite circle. Distension of the stomach brings into action the chemical messengers which send signals of satiety to the appetite centre in the brain. But with bran, this action is short-lived. The analysing and sampling mechanisms in the duodenum which assess the ingested food for nutritional quality soon detect that what is filling the stomach is not food and biofeedback signals report the fact to the brain. So the appetite circle remains open. In animal experiments it has been demonstrated that when rats were given their normal food mixed with bran, they increased their food intake in perfect proportion to the amount of bran that had been added.

The *F-Plan Diet* in fact achieves its results because it is basically a low-calorie diet. The author says, 'Don't count calories. Just follow the menus. The calories are already counted for controlled weight loss.' The menus are, in fact, made up to a choice of 1000 calories, 1250 calories and 1500 calories. It is this factor alone and not the bran that is responsible for the weight loss achieved by the diet.

The Cambridge Diet was published in the USA in 1983, though the diet itself had been propagated by advertisements and mail order since 1980. At 300–600 calories, it is the nearest to total starvation of all the 'big five' diets. It, too, is a new version of an older diet, being in direct line of descent from the infamous liquid protein diet published by the osteopath Robert Linn in his book *The Last Chance Diet,* that appeared in the United States in 1975. The Linn Diet was a liquid formula diet manufactured from beef hides and sow underbelly. Thus the resulting protein, called 'Prolinn', was mainly collagenous protein, which has a very low nutritional value, similar to gelatin, which, as long ago as the early 19th century, was found insufficient to sustain life in animal experiments, being deficient in some of the essential amino acids. *The Last Chance Diet* was published with the usual disclaimer – that it should only be followed under a physician's guidance – and dieters were advised to take vitamin and mineral supplements while on the diet. The Last Chance Diet led to 60 sudden deaths in previously healthy people who followed the diet without medical supervision, and probably lasting physical damage to countless others, before it was finally discredited. It has since been dubbed in medical journals 'the liquid protein mayhem'.

Like the Last Chance Diet, the Cambridge Diet claims to be 'protein sparing', that is, it induces fat loss only while conserving the lean body mass. There is actually no such thing as a protein-sparing diet – the Linn Diet had promised the same safeguard, but at post mortem examination, many of the dieters who had died were found to have severely depleted heart muscle. The claim that the Cambridge Diet is protein-sparing has been discredited in the medical journals. Using the same diet in 11 patients over a period of four weeks, Drs Wilson and Lambert reported in 1979 in the *American Journal of Clinical Nutrition* that there had been a significant loss of nitrogen from their bodies, signifying an appreciable amount of protein loss from muscle.

The book by Dr Alan Howard, *The Cambridge Diet,* published in the USA in 1983, was heavily publicized with three-page advertisements in *Time* and *Newsweek* announcing 'a new scientific breakthrough that works faster and is more effective than you ever thought possible'. It was, of course, no scientific breakthrough – with its extremely low-calorie content the diet *would* work faster, but at a high cost in health and well-being.

The creator of the diet, Dr Alan Howard, claims to be 'a former fatty' who has slimmed himself down with his own diet. He had devised the regime in England but, according to his book, failed to get backing to launch it and went to America, where, he says, the Californian owner of a health club chain provided the two million dollars necessary to get it off the ground. The diet is not available in the shops but is marketed like Avon and Tupperware through local 'counsellers' who give guidance and support to the dieters.

The Cambridge Diet Plan is a 300–600 calorie diet. Its main source of protein is skimmed milk which, though an improvement on Prolinn, is still of low-grade nutritional value. Irrespective of the quality of the dietary protein used, it has been found that all very low-calorie diets produce protein loss from the body. Even if the diet is used as directed for no more than four weeks, small losses of protein are sufficient to create a hazard if they occur in critical organs such as the heart. There is also the danger that some dieters will continue for longer periods than the specified time and could thus be at greater risk. Though Cambridge Plan International makes the usual disclaimer, suggesting a doctor's advice be sought by would-be dieters, the presence of the counsellers who form an efficient network operating up and down the country would to many people seem to render medical advice superfluous.

As reported in the *Journal of the American Medical Association* (25 November 1983) the US Food and Drug Administration had, by 20 December 1982, received 138 complaints of illness, including six reports of death, in people using the Cambridge Diet. In the spring of 1980, the US Postal Service filed suit against Cambridge Plan International on the grounds of misleading claims in its mail-order sales. The suit was settled by a consent decree in which Cambridge International agreed to incorporate the one-month warning statement on product labels, and only since then has this time limit been advised.

The Cambridge Diet was condemned in the *Journal of the American Medical Association* as having 'an unacceptable risk-benefit ratio'. It was recommended that if these very low-calorie diets are used at all, it should be under hospital supervision, with frequent monitoring of blood pressure, mineral salt levels, uric acid levels, and assessment of cardiac function by electrocardiography, with symptomatic treatment of orthostatic hypotension (drop in blood pressure on rising from a sitting or lying position), constipation, diarrhoea, headache, dizziness, hair loss and other problems, a formidable list of the complaints that this diet can give rise to. The inference is that the diet converts previously healthy people into patients requiring hospital treatment.

In spite of the apprehensions voiced in American medical circles, the Cambridge Diet recently came to England. Its creator, Dr Alan Howard, launched the British edition of his book in May 1985 'surrounded by vastly reduced former 20-stoners' described by the *Daily Express* as 'all glowing with the zeal of the converted'. Since then, an intense advertising campaign has been instituted in the British press and elsewhere. Already 1,400 counsellers have been appointed.

The product, a powder formula, is sold through these counsellers and a week's supply costs £12. As the basic ingredient is skimmed milk powder, it represents a healthy profit for the manufacturers. In the lucrative business of weight reduction, there are large profits to be made from very modest outlays. Many of the ingredients used in weight-reduction formulas are the discarded by-products of other industries – bran from milling, skimmed milk from the dairy industry. The beef hides used in the Linn diet were by-products of the meat industry. These discards from other industries, of nominal market value, are retailed to the public as costly weight-reducing formulas.

The weight-reduction industry has become very big business indeed. With the sales of formula products, bran, exercise equipment, the proliferation of weight-reduction clinics and health farms, the publication of books and magazines, the profits are estimated to exceed ten billion dollars a year. The consequent pressures from the industry on women are enormous and have turned many into compulsive dieters.

Other pressures are generated by the health industry. A major pressure has arisen from a section of the medical profession who, in the past decade, have launched a crusade against overweight as a major cause of ill health and one of the risk factors for heart disease. It has now been recognized that this advice was overzealous. Large population studies such as the Framingham Study have revealed that none of the so-called 'risk factors', including obesity, was found to correlate with the degree of morbidity and mortality in the populations concerned. Moderate obesity has now been exonerated as a cause of ill health. The real culprit is the obsessive and continuous drive to combat it by drastic calorie restriction.

3
The new formula

Extensive research over the last several decades has failed to shed any light on the problem of why some people remain lean no matter how much they eat, while others eat sparingly and yet are fat.

It has failed because the fundamental approach has been focused on the simplistic energy input/energy output equation. The answers have been sought in food intake or energy expenditure via exercise. What happens to the food in the body and how the body deals with it in relation to energy utilization and regulation of body build has been ignored entirely. The focus has been on these artificial manipulations of energy balance instead of on the natural laws which govern its generation and utilization.

The answer lies in the understanding of nature's way of dealing with food and how it converts it into energy while at the same time maintaining a stable body weight. When you have understood how the body does this, you will be able to regularize your weight. You will be shown how the body itself has the answers to the mystery. You will be shown how diet and exercise are irrelevant and how the body always overrules these artificial manipulations.

The body regulates food intake in relation to its energy needs through the interplay of two dominant systems, the system which regulates intake and that which regulates energy dispersal.

The internal systems which regulate food input are complex but self-regulatory, subscribed to by complicated neurochemical systems. You will be shown the opiate systems as representative of the various systems which finally regulate food intake.

The energy dispersal mechanism is also self-regulatory. It, too, is composed of numerous interacting systems. You will be shown the action of the brown fat as representative of the energy dispersal systems.

These two phenomena will explain to you many hitherto unsolved paradoxes in weight regulation, as in the case, for instance of twins, both eating the same food, of whom one becomes obese and the other does not. The paradox is that the twin who actually eats less is the one who becomes obese.

They will explain to you the contradiction in the fact that some people leading active working lives eat sparingly yet put on weight. When they go on holiday, these people reduce their activities to the minimum and eat large meals, yet during these holidays they lose weight year after year.

Overweight, healthy people fall into two broad categories. There is one group of people who cannot stop eating. Though they eat substantial meals, they are never satisfied and crave food constantly, eating frequent snacks between meals. They do this in spite of determined efforts to reduce their intake and come to believe, or are made to believe, that they are lacking in will-power. This judgement is misplaced. There is a physical cause for this eating pattern. The excess appetite is caused by physiological factors rather than greed or indiscipline. This pattern of overweight we will call Category A.

The other main group (Category B) have the opposite problem. They eat sparingly and yet put on weight. These people have the greatest difficulty in convincing their doctors that they really do eat very little. Many are greeted with frank disbelief or are made to feel that they are either lying or cheating. They are given the standard advice to eat even less than their already low intake.

The understanding of the opiate systems and the energy dispersal systems represented by the brown fat will give the answer to both these problems.

The natural opiates in the body were discovered in 1975. They have similar properties to morphine with a similar chemical structure, but their potency is estimated to be fifty times that of morphine. The bulk of the peripheral opiates are in the gut nerve cells. The central opiates are situated in the appetite regulatory centre in the brain. Between the two groups, food intake is automatically regulated, regardless of the diet eaten. When food is ingested, opiates from the gut are released, setting up a chain of chemico-electrical reactions. After sufficient numbers are released, the cerebral appetite 'switch-off' mechanism is activated to inhibit further eating.

The inhibition of eating occurs regardless of what you eat or of how much you eat. It is solely dependent on opiate release. You can eat a large amount of food without activating this release, and you can achieve a large opiate release with a much smaller intake. You will be shown how you can activate these natural opiates whenever you wish. Once the opiates are released, the second group of opiates in the brain are automatically activated and the satiety phenomenon is produced. Not only is further eating inhibited, there is physical warmth, emotional tranquillity, and mood uplift.

Once the gut opiates are sufficiently activated, they must bring down the abnormally raised appetite centre to its normal setting. Loss of the capacity to activate the opiates is the main reason why some people crave food all day long and nibble constantly in spite of strenuous efforts to control their intake. Their appetite is never satisfied no matter how much they eat. Their appetite setting has become defective.

When the capacity to release opiates is lost or diminished, the satiety phenomenon cannot occur. The appetite remains unsatisfied no matter how much food is eaten and how much control is exerted. This is the main reason why those in Category A are compelled to eat large meals and constantly eat between meals. It is not a lack of discipline but a defect in the appetite setting brought about by their inability to release sufficient opiates.

The second group of overweights, those in Category B, are those who, in spite of a small food intake, put on weight because of their inability to activate their brown fat to a sufficient degree to dissipate energy. Some of those in Category A may also have this problem in addition to their heavy intake, and there is often a considerable overlap between the two categories.

Brown fat is a special fat located in small quantities in certain sites on the body, mostly in a small area between the shoulder blades, in the chest and in the nape of the neck. Its composition is biologically different from ordinary fat and its function is fundamentally different. Its innervation is also different from that of ordinary white fat. Brown fat is predominantly supplied by the sympathetic nervous system which, when stimulated, causes it to burn calories, regardless of their source. White fat is predominantly innervated by the parasympathetic nervous system. White fat is a storage depot only, storing energy as fat. Brown fat has the opposite function. It burns energy and depletes fat.

Brown fat has the property of generating heat in conditions of cold – the 'thermogenic effect'. It does this by burning calories at a faster rate than the rest of the body.

Brown fat burns up calories at a rate significantly faster

than other bodily cells, producing extra heat. When this heat is not required to raise the body temperature, it is dissipated, ultimately leading to fat depletion.

As with opiate release, brown fat can also be stimulated by food ingestion. In this case, there is no requirement to raise the body temperature. Therefore the heat generated by brown fat activity is dissipated. Brown fat is thus an important factor in burning off any calories ingested in excess of the body's needs, and is an important component of the body's capacity for inherent weight control.

When brown fat activity is defective, people put on weight and remain overweight in spite of eating little. These are the Category B overweights. They are overweight because they are slow burners.

But brown fat can be revitalized by natural means and the weight imbalance redressed. You will be shown not only how you can revitalize the brown fat, but how to regenerate it also.

Insufficient activity of the opiates or brown fat nervous circuits, or a combination of both, results in obesity. Both the opiate and brown fat systems are linked with food ingestion. Their nervous circuits can be activated by a trigger connected with food ingestion. When the appropriate trigger activates both systems simultaneously, the opiates and brown fat not only contribute to weight loss individually, they work in harmony to compound weight loss. They do so by the interaction of the parasympathetic and the sympathetic nervous systems.

In chronic dieting, the opiate systems and the brown fat systems and their intertwined role in controlling energy utilization and body weight become dislocated. Ultimately the weight-control mechanism is itself disrupted.

Brown fat is inactivated during fasting or dieting as an adaptive compensatory measure to conserve the body's energy needs. It is inactivated during vigorous exercise as part of the same conservation process. If the brown fat remains inactivated for too long, as in prolonged dieting, it can atrophy and become unresponsive to stimulation by the usual means. This is why fat people often find it difficult to adapt to cold. The brown fat thermogenic effect is inoperative. Inactivation of the brown fat by dieting is the reason why so many women, who do not actually need to lose weight but decide to do so to follow fashion, become really overweight and set on a course that leads from one diet to another until they finish up with an intractable weight problem.

Other factors can inactivate the brown fat. The thyroid supplements misguidedly given by some diet clinic doctors can do it, again as part of the body's compensatory adaptations to conserve energy.

Brown fat is inactivated during pregnancy, so that the rapidly changing energy requirements of the growing fetus can be accommodated. Many women who have had perfect weight control all their lives begin to put on weight after having children for this reason. They try to regain their pre-pregnant figure too rapidly by dieting, so never manage to get their brown fat activated again after the pregnancy is over. If dieting is not resorted to, the brown fat becomes reactivated at the physiologically right time and at the right pace. Pre-pregnancy weight naturally returns.

Only you can be the proper judge of what your ideal weight should be. The existing ideal body weight tables were derived from insurance company statistics on health and longevity. They were thus based on a biased sample of the community. It has now been recognized that people taking out life insurance are an unrepresentative sample of the community. Additionally, many people, knowing the importance attached to weight by the insurance companies, supply figures considerably less than their true weights. The Metropolitan Life Insurance figures, which for many years provided the standard reference tables, have recently been found to be unrealistically low, and the medical experts have upgraded them to a more realistic level. Yet the currently available diet books still contain these old tables. Many people not originally overweight at all, but who were led to believe from these tables that they were, started the upward spiral of weight gain from going on one of the diets prescribed in these books.

The pinch test, which measures the area between a pinch of the upper arm to gauge the depth of fat, is more individual than weight scales and in that sense more realistic. But the figure of three-quarters of an inch, regarded as the norm, is arbitrary and allows for no variation of individual make-up.

The ideal weight of any individual can only be individually assessed. There is only one you. You are unique and cannot be compared. Your face reflects your weight. When there is more weight than the ideal, your face appears bloated. When there is less than the ideal, it appears hollowed.

Your ideal weight is that at which there is neither bloating nor hollowing around eyes and cheeks and your face is looking at its most attractive. This is the real criterion.

There are wide variations in ideal weight between people of the same height and age. There can be a difference of as much as 20 pounds. You yourself are the best judge of what your ideal weight should be.

It is only the artificial pressures of the fashion industry that have created the picture of the thin, rakish woman that is the ideal in the West today. To the fashion industry, it is the clothes that matter. The women underneath are of secondary importance. Rounded women do not make good clothes horses; they are actually in competition with the clothes themselves. In other parts of the world a rounded female body is considered highly attractive and desirable. In other ages, too, the ideal of feminine beauty was rounded and curvaceous as contemporary paintings show.

Curves are one of the features that distinguish men from women. Women have more fat and fat cells than men. In the average male, fat constitutes up to 10 per cent of body weight. In women it is 24 per cent, the number of fat cells being double that of the male. The higher fat ratio of women to men is brought about by the female sex hormones which come into operation at puberty to produce the feminine curves that begin to appear at this time. This has biological importance as well as aesthetic value in preparing the woman for her maternal role. So a rounded body is very much a feminine attribute. It is invariably well-rounded women who are featured in the centrefold pages of men's magazines.

Fat is the mainstay of bodily contours. No other substance will provide the curves which round the figure. Fat fills the skeletal hollows, the eye sockets, the neck, the elbows, the fingers. The skeleton changes little with age, but when fat is lost, age sets in. If there is insufficient fat in the framework the body will sag. If there is insufficient fat under the skin it will sag and wrinkle.

Body fat is synonymous with the look of youth.

Body fat is synonymous with the functions of youth.

To decide your ideal weight, you must ignore the commercial pressures and the dictates of the fashion industry, and the obsolete weight tables that still figure in the diet books. Only you can decide your ideal weight. You are unique. You have your own build and body make-up. No one else can decide it for you.

But whatever you decide you will be able to achieve it.

The Manorama Formula will explain to you the mechanics
of weight control. The Manorama Formula will show you
how to control the mechanics. You will learn how to
operate the formula skilfully, naturally and appropriately
to regain your ideal weight.

Over the last 15 years every woman and man who was
taught the principle regained their desired weight easily
and naturally, and retained it permanently thereafter.
There was 100 per cent success by this natural method.

So it will be with you. You will have weight control.
This was the promise.

4
No food is fattening

When I told you that you will lose weight without dietary restriction of any sort, I meant it quite literally. You will be able to eat as much as you like, whenever you like. You will be able to eat whatever you like, and this includes all those foods usually forbidden by reducing diets. It includes those currently under a cloud as presumptive causes of ill-health.

Throughout life, much of our attention is inevitably focused on our diet and often our own natural inclinations and food preferences are in conflict with the advice we are given on the nutritional value and health-giving properties of various foods. This advice, too, is constantly changing; food substances are continuously being evaluated and re-evaluated and often these assessments are made on scientifically dubious premises. When in turn they become the subject of lobbying by pressure groups, their true merits and demerits are lost sight of.

For no scientifically established reason, some foods have been credited with special health-giving qualities while others are condemned as harmful and unhealthy. Substitutes for the 'unhealthy' foods are then commercially promoted or are adopted by well-meaning enthusiasts ever ready to take up any new food fad prematurely before it is adequately scientifically evaluated.

In time, attitudes change and foodstuffs once unfashionable become fashionable once more. In the meantime, pressures and confusions are created. The food industry urges you to eat more, the slimming industry to eat less. The food industry promotes one particular food, the diet industry tells you to avoid it and to substitute their own product. Both are often in conflict with your own natural desires and preferences.

The health professionals themselves are subject to fashions and enthusiasms. They have, in the past, condemned many foods since proved innocent, and have overvalued others of poor nutritional value. There is, too, an overlap between the two interests – the commercial and the medical – as many hospital and university research departments receive substantial financial contributions from the food industry.

You will be able to ignore these pressures and gain a true perspective when you know the background of how some foods came to be condemned and others promoted beyond their true value.

Salt was one of the first important foodstuffs to suffer from the vagaries of nutritional fashion. A valued substance for centuries, even used as currency for bartering, it was, a decade ago, condemned as being a cause of high blood pressure (hypertension). The theory had arisen from poorly controlled studies performed earlier this century which have since been invalidated.

A major study specifically performed to establish a correlation or otherwise between salt intake and hypertension, undertaken by Laragh and his co-workers in 1983, conclusively proved that salt intake has no relation to high blood pressure. The addition of excess salt to the diet of a large number of subjects with normal blood pressure failed to produce any rise in pressure after several weeks on the regime.

Additionally, studies of whole communities or even countries have also demonstrated that salt is not conducive to hypertension. High salt eaters, as in south Japan, for instance, have no increased incidence of high blood pressure. Other studies in the United States, Wales,

New Zealand and Sweden have consistently failed to show any difference in sodium intake between normal and hypertensive people.

It has now been established by well-controlled studies that in only one special group of hypertensives identified as 'salt sensitive hypertensives', who represent a minute fraction of the population, does reducing salt intake succeed in bringing down blood pressure. Salt sensitive hypertension has no bearing either on other types of hypertensives or on the normal population.

Salt (sodium chloride) is a natural constituent of the body, of which 80 per cent is made up of saline solution. It is the basis of the essential secretions and has an important role to play in the regulation of the water balance in the tissues. The mechanism by which it does this is a finely tuned system with many checks and balances. The body has a highly efficient regulatory system which assesses its salt requirements and discards the surplus which is then excreted harmlessly in the urine.

Salt is essential for nerve conduction, which operates by the interchange of sodium and potassium ions across the nerve cell membrane. Too little salt can be a serious threat to health. Deaths from dehydration and so-called sunstroke are caused by salt loss from excess sweating. 'Stoker's cramp' arises from the same condition and is treated by salt tablets.

Eliminating salt from the diet will not lower blood pressure. Blood pressure itself has been treated as an undesirable condition in recent years. It is actually part of a highly complex and efficient mechanism, one of the adaptive processes of the body for maintaining an adequate circulation to every organ of the body in every circumstance. Extra exertion, for instance, will produce a rise to ensure an increased supply of blood to heart and muscles. When the ability to increase blood pressure in these circumstances is lost, as in certain rare diseases, dizziness and faintness arise from change of posture from a sitting to a standing position. The current attitude of 'the lower the better' has resulted in regarding anything which lowers the pressure even from perfectly normal levels, such as a low-calorie diet, for instance, meeting with medical approval.

The proven innocence of salt as a cause of high blood pressure has not yet percolated through to the general public. Popular media articles and even health education bodies are still propagating the old dogma, causing many people to eat tasteless, insipid meals in the belief that they are improving their health or reducing their weight.

Like salt, sugar also became unpopular a few decades ago. Substantial health problems were assigned to sugar consumption. Wide and wild allegations were made. Sugar was called the 'sweet poison'. Diabetes, heart disease, obesity and tooth decay were attributed to excess sugar intake. None of these charges have stood the test of time. Now even diabetics are being allowed concentrated sugar substances.

Dietary intake of sugar does not cause diabetes. Diabetes is a metabolic defect of insulin release – a disease affecting a nominal proportion of the population. In normal health, the blood sugar level remains stable within a normal range, regardless of how much sugar is consumed. Whether the diet is sugar-free or sugar-loaded, the body has self-regulatory mechanisms to keep blood sugar levels within the narrow confines of the normal range.

There is no connection between sugar consumption as such and obesity. Neither has any direct link ever been established between sugar intake and heart disease, and in recent years the focus has shifted away from sugar in this context.

Dental caries was the one condition which was directly linked with sugar intake, though even this link was tenuous. The sugar-caries hypothesis was re-examined by Dr R. Cohen in 1979. Writing in the *Proceedings of the Royal Society of Medicine,* the conclusion he drew was that, 'Diet is not the whole story and advocating the exclusion of sugar, even with evangelistic fervour, will not bring about the conquest of caries.' His views were endorsed by Dr W.J. Darby, writing in the *Journal of Clinical Periodontology* of the same year, who categorically stated, 'The current narrow focus on reduction of sucrose in the diet is not defensible.' A timely editorial in the *American Journal of Clinical Nutrition* (July 1983) reminds us that, 'No large-scale studies on the effect of sugar restriction have yet demonstrated subsequent meaningful falls in dental caries.' Neither have any such studies been reported since the time of his report. On the other hand, evidence from sugar-cane-producing communities that use sugar and sugar-loaded sweets as prime sources of energy supplementation from an early age demonstrates a significant freedom from tooth decay.

Sugar is natural to the body. The bulk of ingested food converts to sugar before it can be taken up by the body as its main source of energy. It is a concentrated source of energy, the first line of defence in shock, debility and depression. Attempted suicides are given high-concentration sugar drinks to lift their depression.

In health, the body is equipped to regulate its sugar intake with precision. It indicates its needs through the desirability factor. Need for ready energy is expressed by a craving for sweet substances; surfeit is indicated by revulsion. These are the only true criteria for judging the correct intake of sugar.

The indictment of dietary fat as a cause of heart disease has arisen largely from a paper published by Professor A.

Keys in 1968, published in the medical journal *Circulation*, in which he propounded the theory that a high dietary intake of fat was responsible for the rising incidence of coronary heart disease in Western countries. Keys selected data from World Health Organization tabulations gained from six countries to reach this conclusion. Dr George Mann, of Vanderbilt University Medical School, has recently reviewed this paper and has pointed out its obvious defects. Of all the countries in the world only six were selected. Variables independent of dietary fat which could equally well have been contributory factors were ignored. So the 'diet-heart' hypothesis was based on epidemiological data gained from this one study. Subsequently, data gathered on a similar basis from numerous countries produced results which did not accord with those of Professor Keys. There are many instances of populations consuming extremely high fat intakes – the Eskimos, the Masai tribes of Africa, or the llamas of Tibet, who have a very low incidence of heart and circulatory disease. Nor can the hypothesis be sustained in countries like Sweden, Israel and Switzerland, which have a high incidence of coronary heart disease and low fat intakes.

Dr Mann described how the 'diet-heart' hypothesis – the theory that dietary fat causes coronary heart disease – had snowballed from Keys' paper: 'In a few years some combination of the urgent needs of health agencies, oil-food companies and ambitious fat scientists had transformed that fragile hypothesis into treatment dogma', he said. The results were predictable: 'The dietary dogma was a money-maker for segments of the food industry, a fund raiser for the Heart Association and busy work for thousands of fat chemists.'

Since Keys' paper, cholesterol has been written about

as a dangerous foreign substance. In fact, it is a normal and important constituent of the body. It is the precursor of the bile acids and of the steroid hormones, including the sex hormones. Only 10–20 per cent of the body's total cholesterol is actually obtained from ingested food; if fat intake is insufficient to make up the remainder, the body reacts by increasing the rate of synthesis. In one study, a patient on a low-cholesterol diet made up by synthesis milligram for milligram exactly the amount deducted from his diet. Others made up nearly the exact amount.

In normal health, the homeostatic mechanisms of the body function efficiently to keep blood levels of cholesterol within the normal range. As with sugar metabolism, delicate and precise systems of checks and balances via feed-back mechanisms ensure that blood cholesterol is kept at a constant level with little day to day variation. A small number of people, accounting for a minute proportion of the population, have a hereditary disease called hypercholesterolaemia, in which the body's handling of fat metabolism is defective, and in these people the blood cholesterol levels are raised and they do have a higher incidence of heart disease. In a few other conditions, such as thyroid disease, blood fat levels are raised as a secondary effect. The oral contraceptive ('the pill') also slightly raises the blood fat levels. But in none of these conditions is dietary fat responsible.

The 'diet-heart' hypothesis rests on the simplistic proposition that the level of fats in the blood is directly proportionate to the amount of fat ingested in the diet. That this is simplistic and incorrect was conclusively demonstrated by the important Tecsumeh Study carried out in 1976 by the Department of Epidemiology of Ann Arbor Medical School in the United States. The study, conducted among a large section of the town of Tecsumeh, attempted to correlate the fats consumed the previous day with the blood fat levels the following day. There was no correlation between the two. The blood fat levels were found to be quite independent of any dietary constituent and independent of the amounts of fat ingested.

The Tecsumeh study made another significant observation. In the population examined, there was no correlation between the blood fat levels and whether the fat ingested the previous day was saturated or unsaturated. Thus another facet of the 'diet-heart' hypothesis, that saturated, i.e. animal, fat is the main culprit in causing heart disease, while polyunsaturated fats (fats of vegetable origin) are innocent, was invalidated.

Since Keys' original paper in 1953, research has been conducted mainly on experimental animals, the rabbit having been chosen as the most convenient for the purpose. These creatures were fed large amounts of cholesterol in their diets. But the rabbit is a herbivorous animal to whom dietary fat is foreign, and these experiments are flawed on that account alone – the changes in the blood vessels the diet produced were considered by many critics as being consistent with an allergic reaction to an alien diet.

In recent years, however, the results of long-term, large-scale human population intervention studies conducted over several years are gradually becoming available. Of those available to date, the Framingham Study in the United States, the Israel Ischaemic Heart Disease Study, the MRFIT Study, the WHO European Study, the North Karelia Study, and the Lipid Research Clinics Study, in fact all the large-scale studies made to date, have all demonstrated no difference in mortality and morbidity between those who had lowered their fat intake and those consuming an ordinary diet, or those consuming predominantly unsaturated fat from those eating saturated. Attempts have been made to explain away these results, but their consistency and uniformity have seriously undermined the 'diet-heart' hypothesis, and research is now moving on to the search for other factors, such as abnormalities in the clotting mechanism in the blood, or to genetic research which would identify more precisely those at risk of coronary heart disease. These facts also have not percolated through to the general public, and warnings about the dangers of cholesterol and of saturated fat are still being disseminated by health education bodies and the media.

The final conclusions of the National Academy of Sciences and the National Research Council of America, described as 'the supreme court of science', published as far back as 1980, which found that no prevention of coronary heart disease could be achieved by dietary control of cholesterol, should have decided the issue. In England, the best-known and most influential reports, those of the National Advisory Committee on Nutrition Education (NACNE) and of the Committee on Medical Aspects of Food Policy (COMA), have been widely misinterpreted as supporting the diet-heart hypothesis. In fact, in neither is there any assertion that fats in the diet are responsible for coronary heart disease in the population as a whole. The COMA report categorically states about cholesterol, 'We believe that current intake is not excessive and that evidence for an influence of this level of intake on blood cholesterol is inconclusive.' On reduction of the saturated unsaturated fat ratio in the diet, the report admits that multiple-risk factor intervention trials 'have not shown convincing evidence of benefit.' Their recommendations on reducing fat intake were actually directed only at those at increased risk of coronary heart disease, i.e. those with a strong family history of the disease or those with familial hypercholesterolaemia or their close relatives.

The NACNE report (1983) stated: 'Given the variation in current scientific opinion, the limitation of dietary cholesterol should not be incorporated as a key feature of the dietary advice for the UK.'

Nevertheless, both the COMA and NACNE reports were widely interpreted by the media and disseminated to the public as indications for the reduction of dietary fats in the whole population. Every day some new recommendation from some well-meaning public body brings out a new version of the old formula – less cholesterol, and a higher ratio of polyunsaturated to saturated fat.

The prohibition against red meat is founded on 'the hidden danger' lurking within it – the minute quantity of cholesterol it contains, and a higher proportion of saturated to non-saturated fat. The virtues of polyunsaturated fat, which in essence means margarine and cooking fats made of linseed or other vegetable oil instead of animal fat, are high on the list of enthusiasms of what Professor Sir John McMichael, who examined the alleged properties of polyunsaturated fat very thoroughly, calls the 'polyunsaturated fat evangelists.' The polyunsaturated fat theory arose from foundations as shaky as those of the cholesterol hypothesis itself. There is no evidence whatever that it will prevent heart disease. In Israel, which consumes twice as much polyunsaturated fat as most Western countries, there is a very high incidence of coronary heart disease. On the contrary, there is evidence that polyunsaturated fats double the incidence of gallstones, and they have recently been implicated in some studies as being responsible for a higher incidence of cancer. The saturated fat scare has caused unnecessary limitations in diet and caused unnecessary anxiety in the public.

Without sufficient ingested fat, the body is unable to utilize the fat-soluble vitamins, such as A, D, E and K. It is estimated that one million children a year go blind in Asia, not only because of insufficient vitamin A in their diet, but because only a part of it is absorbed due to a lack of fat in their food.

Prohibitions on red meat and dairy food are not only based on misconception, they can be actively harmful. Animal products are the only source of Vitamin B12. Complete vegans (those who eschew all animal products) run the risk of pernicious anaemia. They may take supplements of the vitamin but these are poorly absorbed from the gastrointestinal tract. Children raised as vegans have a lower height and weight than those on a normal diet and suffer other health problems.

There is no danger of eating too much fat. As with salt, our own internal assessors are the surest safeguard against this. Any fat ingested over and above the body's needs brings about revulsion and subsequent aversion. Thereby the intake is very accurately measured. Nature has, in fact, produced its own mechanism for ensuring a healthier, balanced diet. Ill-founded food strictures prescribe dietary habits inappropriate to the body's needs and lead to imbalance in food intake leading to other health problems.

No food is inherently bad. The only bad food is decomposed food. Cooking fat is harmful when the same fat is used over and over again and the carbonated fats have accumulated. Under no other circumstances are fats harmful in themselves.

The two main considerations in selecting foods are purity and relative nutritional value. Animal fat is superior to vegetable because of its vitamin content. Vegetable and fruit fibre has less nutritional value than the pulp. White sugar has more concentrated nutrients than brown. Bran has no food value whatsoever.

In following the Manorama Formula, you will not be asked to eat bran. Bran is a non-food. There is no known human enzyme capable of digesting it. Bran has no health-giving properties whatsoever. Neither has it any weight-reducing properties. It actually has some actively harmful qualities.

Bran is a by-product of the milling industry, the tough outer protective covering of the grain, husks that have been rejected by every community in the world. Even animals fed these husks in their food in the third world reject them. From time immemorial every primitive community has developed its own crude milling methods for getting rid of this indigestible husk. A simple experiment with a grain of wheat will tell you at once that it is inedible.

The cult of adding bran to the Western diet grew out of the fibre hypothesis originated by Dr Denis Burkitt in the late 1960s. He found that relatively few rural Africans suffered from colon cancer and other gut disorders. These rural communities, in common with most third world communities, live largely on crudely milled grain and the available locally grown food. Burkitt's theory was that the rapid passage of bowel contents caused by high-fibre diets allowed less time for cancer-inducing agents to form and additionally lowered the concentration of any potential carcinogen.

This presupposes that food has the potentiality for becoming carcinogenic in the gut. There is no evidence that food in transit undergoes any carcinogenic change, or provokes a carcinogenic reaction in the gut cells. Neither is there evidence that rapid transit decreases the risk of cancer formation. The fibre theory was therefore not only evidentially unsupported, but disproved in practice by later studies. These studies showed that when black Africans who migrated to the towns and adopted the diet of urban whites with a lower fibre content, they continued to have a low incidence of colon cancer. Further, this immunity extended to the second generation of black Africans living in towns. Other studies have shown that there are other communities in the world who also have a low incidence of colon cancer but who consume the average low-fibre Western diet – the Mormons of Utah, for example – a fact that cannot be explained by Burkitt's theories.

These later findings received little publicity, however, and Burkitt meanwhile extensively propagated his theory in the West, speaking at many medical meetings, and it caught the imagination of the media. Though Burkitt's theory had been refuted, very soon 'all the diseases of Western civilization' began to be attributed to lack of dietary fibre. Because bran, though inedible, is all fibre, it was promoted by commercial interests as a valuable food. It had the advantage that it was a discarded by-product of the milling industry and of low commercial value. So almost overnight, this low-cost substance was turned into a highly priced profit-maker.

As we have seen, Burkitt's theory rested on the alleged beneficial effects of rapid intestinal transit of the bowel contents produced by the greater residual bulk of a high-fibre diet. In fact, the body has its own highly efficient mechanisms for moving the bowel contents at the pace most conducive to the effective metabolization of its nutrients. The entire absorption of these nutrients takes place through the gut wall, a process which takes some time. Therefore, an unnaturally rapid passage of bowel contents reduces the absorption of nutrients. The minerals and the vitamins A, D, E and K are largely absorbed through the lower gut, the area which suffers most from unnatural rapid transit. Recent studies in the *American Journal of Clinical Nutrition* have demonstrated serious depletion of these substances in subjects adding bran to their diet. Additionally, bran produces serious side effects of its own – it produces phytic acid, which depletes the body of zinc, iron and calcium, all important nutritional elements whose role cannot be performed by any other elements.

Fibre has been found to cause disturbance of the normal gut flora. Since it is indigestible, bran ferments in the gut, causing abnormal noxious gases and producing distension and flatulence. This fermentation can even cause obstruction.

On the basis of all the major studies made on both sides of the Atlantic, therefore, over the last decade, the facts, as they appear in the actual reports and before reinterpretation, appear to be as follows:

Sugar restriction is only necessary in the case of diabetics, who amount to less than 2 per cent of the population.

Salt restriction is only of benefit to salt-sensitive hypertensives, who number only a minute fraction of all cases of hypertension and form an infinitesimal percentage of the population at large.

Fat restriction, whether saturated or polyunsaturated, is applicable only to cases of familial hypercholesterolaemia and other diseases in which raised blood cholesterol is a secondary symptom, in all amounting to less than 0.2 per cent of the population.

The distinction between the benefits of saturated and polyunsaturated fat is a theoretical concept only.

The pressure to eat bran is detrimental and has potentially serious consequences.

In the normal, healthy population, therefore, pressures to eat bran and strictures against sugar, salt and fat are biologically unsound.

Food is the largest commercial commodity in the world. Food substances are therefore often promoted for commercial reasons distinct from their nutritional value. Thus unnecessary confusions and anxieties are created.

The modern science of nutrition is itself in its infancy. The discovery of vitamins and the recognition of the importance of minerals has occurred only in the last 100 years or so. But from time immemorial mankind has been instinctively making the correct selection of essential nutritional elements by making use of the body's own natural equipment for indicating its biological needs. The body has an in-built mechanism for ensuring that the appropriate nutritional choices are made. You will see that this mechanism is an infallible guide to your food requirements and a far better one than bowing to the pressures of the food industry or reliance on short-lived nutritional fashions.

The greatest weakness of blanket evaluation of foods is the neglect of the environmental conditions in which the individual lives. Climatic conditions affect the individual directly and therefore nutritional needs will vary between people living in hot dry climates and those living in cold wet climates. Climatic conditions affect you indirectly because they determine the food produced in your area.

For this reason, food produced locally is most compatible with the inhabitants of the area. As the seasons change, so the variety of food changes.

When food is at its best, it is most abundant and cheapest. Therefore, the most rational way of selecting food useful to the body's needs is to choose what is personally desirable and cheapest.

5
Exercise – the redundant factor

You are not being asked to exercise to lose weight. Weight loss by exercise is costly, transient and potentially damaging.

Voluntary muscular activity in the course of walking, work or sport is rewarding in itself. But such activities for the purpose of reducing weight are self-defeating.

The exploitation of muscular power in competitive sport has biological value. It served to establish the social hierarchy when man first began living in communities. Muscular activity is both rewarding in itself and in the achievement of its goals. But to advocate it as a means of reducing weight is biologically insupportable.

No particular exercise regime has any reducing virtue in itself. Regardless of the nature of the muscular activity, its intensity and duration, if the energy expended remains within the bounds of the ready energy supply available, body weight will remain unchanged. Energy input and expenditure will be balanced and internal stability maintained.

When, however, muscular activity is imposed without regard to your true status, when the energy expenditure is in excess of energy intake in food, it exhausts the energy supply and becomes a pressure on the system. Weight loss is then achieved at the cost of inner stability and potential abnormal chemical changes. Muscular activity under pressure will be accompanied by altered electrical conduction to the nervous system, changes in the composition of the electrolytes, and production of

toxic end products in the body. These changes will be
reflected in subjective feelings of stress, strain and pain.

Three main areas of ambiguity underline the current
pressures to lose weight and to exercise strenuously.
Firstly, the correlation between a particular weight and
health has never been scientifically established. What the
normal weight for any particular individual is has not
been clinically determined. As we have already seen in
Chapter 3, the previously accepted figures, gained from
insurance company data, have been found to be invalid.
Blanket statements to the effect that 'overweight is
unhealthy', though not scientifically valid, exert insidious
but significant pressure.

Secondly, the view that exercise protects against coronary heart disease, a strongly emotive factor in the pressure
to indulge in high-intensity exercise regardless of personal
status, is dangerous. The claim is based on the fact that
seasoned athletes develop increased cardiovascular and
oxygenating capacity through the opening up of additional
circulatory channels. They are thus able to prolong the
time spent in muscular activity before the onset of the
'pain barrier'. The parallel between seasoned athletes and
those who set out forcibly to 'break the pain barrier' is
not tenable. In the latter, the immediate and remote
risks to health and life are unacceptably high. Significant
numbers of cases of sudden death in young, healthy men
who have disregarded the pain barrier have been reported
over a substantial number of years. Many have dropped
dead playing squash. The same enforced pressures have
precipitated significant numbers of sudden deaths while
jogging.

The third area of ambiguity is the various connotations
applied to the unqualified use of the term 'fitness'. As
used today, the term does not have a biological value but
a commercial one. It is used by commercial interests to

imply that in some way you are less fit than you should be, thus casting unfounded doubts on your abilities. The implications of unfitness create feelings of inferiority and insecurity which are used to good effect in promoting the sale of gadgets and programmes of dubious value. Every healthy person is a fit person and pressures to exercise should be weighed in the balance of the commercial interests involved.

Fitness is now a billion-dollar industry, and its promotion is commensurate with the size of its profitability. Electric treadmills, exercycles, antigravity boots, rowing machines and dumb-bells, aerobic gymnasia and books are a profitable spin-off. Subsidiary industries have emerged supplying warm-up suits, leotards, ankle weights, leg-warmers, fitness shoes and sporting bands. Exercise physiologists, 'individual body-building', personalized development and 'increased body awareness' are some of the additional subsidiary spin-offs in this expanding market.

The combined pressures from the diet industry, the health industry, the fitness industry and, for women, the additional pressures from the fashion industry and latterly the feminist lobby, constantly urge weight loss at whatever cost.

The message from the diet, health and fitness industries is that if you are not thin you are not healthy. The message from the fashion industry is that if you are not thin you are not attractive. The message from the feminist lobby is that women should exercise to develop hard, muscular bodies like those of men, 'to break the "weaker sex" mould' in the effort to achieve physical as well as economic, political and social equality with men. This is an unrealistic aim. In the average young male, 15 per cent of body weight is made up of fatty tissue and 52 per cent of muscle. In the average young woman, the ratio is 27 per cent fat to 40 per cent muscle. This gender ratio is genetically determined and mediated by the sex hormones. There is nothing that can alter it short of administering male hormones, a practice that was carried out some years ago by female athletes until significant side effects such as hirsutism began to appear.

Spurred on by these pressures, attractive, healthy people, believing that they are overweight, unattractive and in some way unhealthy and unfit, have felt it expedient to go to any lengths to achieve the degree of thinness deemèd essential for their health, fitness and looks. Many have run the gamut of diets from the Scarsdale to the Cambridge only to find that they remain the same weight or are even fatter than before. Finally, disillusioned by the time and energy wasted, they have turned to exercise as a last resort.

Weight loss by exhaustive muscular activity is achieved by calorie manipulation. The formula is the same as that in dieting except that it is calorie output rather than calorie intake that is manipulated. The interim chemical changes induced may be different, but the body's reaction will be the same. Whether the weight loss is achieved by workouts, jogging, aerobics, yoga, or exercising on treadmills or exercycles, no matter how long the weight loss is sustained, when the exercise is discontinued the body is programmed to replace the lost weight as rapidly as possible. This rebound weight gain is known in medical circles as the 'retired athlete's syndrome'. This syndrome operates more forcefully when non-athletes resort to exhaustive exercise two or three times a week. The lost weight will be replaced between every session.

In any case, any weight lost by exhaustive exertion will be small in proportion to the amount of effort expended. Theoretically, calorie expenditure by this means should alter the energy equation and cause weight loss through dissipation of calories. In fact, an important factor has been left out of the calculation. In its defence against the extra demands made on it, the body, as an adaptive measure to conserve energy, compensates for the excess expenditure by switching off other energy expending mechanisms. Further, the brown fat is not only temporarily switched off, its prolonged inactivation leads to atrophy from disuse and it eventually becomes less and less responsive to stimulation. Thus, as in dieting, a situation is created whereby it becomes less and less easy to shed excess weight and proportionately more intensive programmes are required to lose the same amount.

Thus weight loss from exercise is comparatively small and achieved at the cost of a reduction in overall capacity to maintain an ideal body weight.

Much of the current pressure towards strenuous exercise has arisen from the fact that it has been promoted for many years as a protective factor against coronary heart disease, while lack of such exercise was indicted as one of the 'risk factors' for the condition. But long-term studies on large populations have failed to support this claim. Out of a total of five major studies carried out to date, four have shown no correlation between either overweight or lack of exercise and coronary heart disease. The fifth, and most recent, the United Kingdom Heart Disease Project, in fact demonstrated a negative correlation. A total of 18,210 men aged between 40 and 59 from 24 different factories took part in the study. One group was given the conventional advice on the benefits of exercise and the hazards of overweight. The other group, the controls, were given no specific advice. After six years, the results were tabulated and, instead of the expected benefits, the doctors monitoring the study found a significantly *higher* cardiovascular morbidity and mortality in the group who had followed their advice on extra exercise and weight reduction compared to the control group who were given no such counselling.

In spite of the risks to health and life, exercise programmes entailing sudden rapid, intensive exertion remain in fashion. The recent promotion of 'aerobics' is part of this trend. Aerobic exercise entails sudden demands on energy in excess of the body's ready supply. One of its advocates, Jane Fonda, exhorts her readers to 'go for the burn' – 'You feel the burn when you have difficulty in contracting that muscle for a moment,' she says. 'It is simply a sign that you are using that muscle vigorously and effectively, working hard and deep.' In fact, what is being asked of you is that you exhaust your ready energy supply and make reckless demands on your reserves.

The proper utilization of sudden mobilization of reserve energy is in emergency situations. In such circumstances adrenaline is released in a master plan to meet the sudden demand for increased energy. Adrenaline causes an immediate rise in the rate of heartbeat and in the force of its contractions. Additionally, it releases extra glucose from the stores in the liver and discharges it into the bloodstream. This is then carried via the increased blood supply to the voluntary muscles at a faster rate to supply their raised energy requirements. By another route, adrenaline increases the rate and depth of breathing to match the oxygen supply with the increased glucose utilization. This adaptive measure is life-saving and the trauma to the system entailed is justified in the right circumstances. The repeated self-inflicted trauma of exhaustive exercise on the other hand, is an unjustifiable demand on the system and an unnecessary risk to health and life.

The term 'aerobics' means oxygen-utilizing. The claim is made that aerobic exercise increases the amount of oxygen in the tissues, which is said to be beneficial. But the fast, strenuous exercise implied by the term aerobics increases the oxygen demands to a point and at a rate where even the adaptive measures described above are unable to meet the demand. On the contrary, aerobics, instead of increasing the oxygenation of the tissues, actually decreases it. Far from having any beneficial effect on the tissues, lactic acid and other toxic metabolites, formed when there is insufficient oxygen to metabolize glucose, are noxious end products of the process.

The rapid heartbeat and faster breathing produced by aerobics is extolled as a desirable condition. In fact, it is using the emergency adaptive mechanisms of the body as a means to an end. Rapid heartbeat and faster breathing to produce additional oxygen utilization even if it were achieved by aerobics, have no advantage. The body measures its oxygen requirements accurately. Its fluctuating needs are appropriately met by physiological mechanisms which alter the respiratory rate according to circumstances. Excess oxygen is not only superfluous, it is as dangerous as a deficit, as was painfully demonstrated in the fifties, when a significant number of babies were rendered blind by the over-enthusiastic use of oxygen in the newborn state.

Additionally, 'breaking through the pain barrier' by means of workouts and aerobics is promoted as a desirable state by its advocates. In fact, stress, strain and pain are signals setting boundaries to the amount of exertion that will be tolerated by the body. Disregarding the boundaries set by these messages can lead to physical injury. A recent major Japanese study cited a 25 per cent incidence of injury among those indulging in exhaustive exercise. Similar high incidences have been reported in the West. Fractures, dislocations, neck and back injuries have been frequent, as have injuries to joints, tendons, ligaments and muscles and, in the case of up-hill joggers, the characteristic bilateral rupture of the Achilles tendons.

The dubious theory of the relationship between exhaustive exercise and fitness has produced a new medical condition, referred to in the *Lancet* as 'the morbid exercise syndrome'. Usually starting as an exercise programme to reduce weight, a kind of obsession takes over the individual whereby he or she cannot stop exercising, even in the presence of physical disability and skeletomuscular injury.

Exercise exhaustive enough to cause weight loss will have other side effects. It has been estimated that impaired reproductive functioning, manifested in amenorrhoea (cessation of the periods), abnormal monthly cycles, including anovulatory cycles and abnormal patterns in the sex hormones, affect as many as 50 per cent of women indulging in these activities, an important factor to be considered in those intending to have families.

The same natural principle applied in the instinct to nourish can be applied to movement also, involving the harmonizing of voluntary activities with the inner signals from the skeletomuscular system. You can have perfect posture, muscle tone and ease of movement without exercise entailing interference with your energy balance, or risk of injury, and they can be achieved naturally and in the ordinary course of the day in keeping with your individual life-style. In following the Manorama Formula your energy balance will not be subjected to sudden demands or artificial manipulations that disrupt your weight regulatory mechanisms, and you will achieve, naturally and effortlessly, permanent and perfect weight control.

6
The scientific basis

The starting point of normalizing the body build/weight control mechanism is the normalization of hunger and appetite.

Unfulfilled hunger/appetite are abnormal. Only when their demands are met can they make their proper contribution to normalizing body build/weight control. When their needs have been fulfilled, they initiate a series of biological processes which correct under or overweight and automatically lead to ideal body weight.

You have an individual ideal weight because you have an individual build. No two people have identical builds. Similarly, no two people have identical hunger/appetite. Within the normal range there are individual variations of the weight/hunger/appetite combination. These detailed individual variations are in keeping with the biological importance of hunger and appetite and the uniqueness of your build.

Biologically, feelings of hunger and appetite are crucial to health and survival. Without hunger/appetite there would be no concept of the need for nourishment. To ensure survival, therefore, there has to be an in-built mechanism independent of other internal factors and environmental conditions, a mechanism which asserts itself with a force which demands response as a priority. There has to be a natural compulsion to eat which will safeguard the well-being of the individual. This mechanism is the subjective sensation of hunger and appetite, coupled with the underlying system of complex feedback processes in the body which give rise to them.

To ensure sustained replenishment of energy, hunger/appetite are linked to the life flow. They become operative at birth and continue throughout life. When they diminish, life diminishes.

Hunger/appetite are vital signals.

Not only are they vital, they are central to the stability of all the systems in the body. Without regular arousal of hunger there would be no means to time the body's energy needs. Its supply would become sporadic. All the systems in the body would then lose their natural rhythm and function at an erratic pace.

Hunger and appetite not only time the body's energy needs, they also measure them. If energy needs were not accurately measured by hunger and appetite, the bodily systems would not only slow down, but some tissues would become permanently damaged when inadequately nourished. Then again, if the food intake were in excess of the energy needs, the surplus would be stored as fat.

Hunger and appetite work hand in hand to determine the bodily needs of the time with a high degree of precision. But they are not identical. It is important to understand the distinction and to realize their value individually and jointly.

Hunger determines the total calorie and fluid requirements of the body.

Appetite takes into account the total number of calories demanded by hunger and helps to select the right distribution of fats, carbohydrates and protein to supply them.

The three main groups of foods – fats, proteins and carbohydrates – all convert to energy in the form of blood sugar. However, they convert to energy at varying rates. If a correct combination is achieved, a steady supply of energy between meals is ensured. Carbohydrates are metabolized earliest and convert to energy first; the proteins follow, and lastly come the fats. Sugar supplies energy almost immediately.

Fats and proteins are not only essential sources of energy, their metabolized end products are necessary to repair and replenish the tissues. Appetite determines the exact amount of fats and proteins required for this specific purpose. It checks this factor with the amount required for energy, and by a sensitive and sophisticated system of measurement, computes the precise figure of total fat and protein requirement.

The appetite's third criterion of selection is concerned with a small but vital quantity of important substances, substances which do not figure in the energy/repair calculation as such but which are, however, essential for the proper functioning of all the bodily systems. These are the vitamins, minerals and electrolytes. The appetite takes these needs into account when making the final optimal selection.

Without hunger there would be no concept of the necessity of eating. Without appetite there would be no indication of the necessary composition of food intake to match the body's vital needs. The correct composition of food intake would be left to chance; it would be a hit or miss affair whether intake fulfilled bodily needs or not. It would be equally hit or miss whether the body was insufficiently nourished or overburdened with an excess of nutrients.

Robust hunger and appetite are indications of health, vitality and vigour. To give them free rein does not represent loss of control as the diet planners would imply. Compliance with their demands is the fundamental basis of individual fulfilment, development and true control.

In dieting, hunger/appetite and the finer tuning of taste are blunted by neglect and confrontation. To vitalize the weight-loss mechanism, hunger and appetite have to be acknowledged and nurtured, and food intake matched to appetite by its taste value.

Hunger and appetite will not make you vulnerable to weight gain. They will not arise to your detriment. They will come into focus precisely at the time most advantageous to you. They will arise at the time when the meal will best serve its purpose, when it will produce energy and satiety, but not fat.

Appetite arises at the appropriate time, almost immediately after the first intimation of hunger. If allowed its options, it will make a perfect selection of the nutrients the body requires at that particular time.

But though appetite emerges after hunger, they both peak at the same time. This peaking is synchronized by an internal clock. There is an individual variation whereby people are most hungry at different times of the day. Diets disregard this individual variation and, by enforcing fixed meals, disturb the natural timing of hunger and appetite and the optimal functioning of the ensuing metabolic processes.

The signals of hunger and appetite arise in accordance with the internal clock. Your clock is special to you. It is not necessarily in keeping with someone else's clock. It is not even in keeping with the external clock. But for you it is the most harmonizing clock and your metabolic status will be indicated by that clock. Food eaten at the time it specifies will convert to energy and will not be stored as fat.

At the peaking of hunger and appetite, your imagination will naturally focus on food. Equally naturally, you should exploit your imagination in choosing the meal you most desire at that particular time.

In the sequence of events brought about by your biological clock, imagination is an important link between the vital instincts of survival and their fulfilment. Imagination helps to identify and seek out the object of instinct fulfilment. Specifically in connection with the instinct to eat, it identifies and seeks out the food items most necessary to the body at that particular time.

Imagination matches available options with past satisfactory experiences. This is instinctive and leads to appropriate choices of food. Imagination matches the bodily needs of the hour with the choices realistically available, taking into account the personal past experiences of the individual, and arriving at the appropriate selection. It will do this instinctively and naturally, provided it is not encumbered by the restraints of fixed diets which are unrelated to the real needs of the body. By dictating rigid menus, reducing diets discount personal imagination, thereby denying its crucial biological role. Diets not only exert physical control but, by eliminating the use of imagination, assert mental control also, which is their most enslaving aspect.

Progressing from the hunger-appetite-imagination sequence, taste is heightened. Taste is the fourth vital component of the body's mechanism to secure an optimally nutritional food intake.

Taste, or personal preference, is based on two considerations: (1) taste acquired from earlier experience, in other words, from a liking for food that has provided satisfaction in the past. This is a valid preference because it has stood the test of time as individually compatible and beneficial; (2) the bodily needs of the time, an equally valid factor.

Taste is a biological asset.

Taste checks food for the finer details such as purity, edibility and appropriateness of temperature. After this preliminary check, the food progresses to the assessors and sensors in the upper part of the gut which analyse it

for its compliance with the hunger-appetite-taste component and double-check its usefulness to the body. During
the course of the meal, the taste for it proportionately
diminishes. When enough has been eaten to satisfy the
body's needs, taste for that particular food or combination
of foods ceases. Thus taste is an important guide to
nutritional requirements and an indicator of when those
needs have been fulfilled.

Hunger/appetite/imagination/taste normally peak simultaneously according to the internal clock. When these
signals and pointers are not properly obeyed, the purpose
of eating is not fulfilled.

Reducing diets contravene these natural demands on
all counts. They dictate non-preferred foods in non-
preferred quantities at non-preferred times. By so doing,
they interfere with the primary purpose of eating.

You have seen in Chapter 1 how a calorie-restricted
diet fails to supply adequate energy, and how lowered
blood sugar leads to the slowing down of all bodily
systems through the slowing down of the basal metabolic
rate. You have also seen how this factor leads to rebound
weight gain.

To make doubly sure that this rebound weight gain is
not interfered with, the weight regulating mechanism
makes its own contribution. It does this by recruiting
additional circuits which interreact with the opiates rather
than the blood sugar, achieving its purpose by maintaining
the setting of the appetite centre in the brain at a
high level, leading to increased intake of food, and by
inhibiting brown fat activity, leading to the conservation
of energy expenditure.

The clockwork precision with which appropriate food
intake is assessed, timed and implemented is primarily to
ensure a ready, steady, and sufficient energy supply to

the body. Intertwined with this objective, and comp-lementary to it, is the maintenance of ideal body weight and build as a base for energy utilization.

The weight-control mechanism computes body weight with the same precision as it does food intake. It computes weight distribution down to the minutest detail and sets it as the norm. When there is a deviation from this norm, the mechanism retains its tendency to return to the norm. The capacity to shift towards the norm comes into force when the food intake has been assessed by the assessors and sensors in the upper part of the gut as being sufficient to meet the nutritional needs of the body. The opiates at the same level of the gut are then released, bringing about the sensation of satiety at the physical, emotional and intellectual level which precludes any incentive to alter the state.

This is dependent on the release of opiates in sufficient amounts at all levels of the body. Only when sufficient numbers of opiates are released is further eating inhibited.

Conversely, if the ingested food does not match the appetite-hunger criterion, then on the one hand an energy imbalance is created and on the other hand appetite is left unsatisfied and continues to exert its demands for further eating.

You were told in Chapter 3 that brown fat has special qualities. These clusters of special cells in various parts of the body are concerned primarily with maintaining a stable body temperature. In a cold environment they produce heat to raise the body temperature in order to maintain it at the normal level regardless of the external cold. These cells, though fat cells, differ from ordinary white fat cells in that they do not store calories. They are entirely concerned with burning calories and turning them into heat. Further, they burn ingested calories at a rate significantly faster than the norm. The brown fat system is the only system that dissipates calories in the form of heat. They are not converted into any other form of energy. They are not stored as fat.

In addition to cold, in the right circumstances brown fat can be stimulated by food ingestion. It then burns calories significantly faster than normal, identical to the cold-stimulus effect. But unlike the thermogenic goal, as this extra heat is not required, it is dissipated at a rapid rate.

Loss of calories via brown fat activity is the only route whereby calories can be lost continuously without being made good. Brown fat activity does not set up any compensatory mechanism to replace those lost calories. When calories are used up in this way, there is no rebound weight gain.

Brown fat can lose calories at a fast rate every time food is ingested. You will be shown that it can also lose calories in-between meals. It can and does so without any compensatory gain.

The brown fat can be compared to a furnace in the body and its fuel to calories. It alone can shed three pounds in weight per week. Unlike reducing diets, this does not lead to lowered blood sugar. It does not raise the appetite. There are none of the adverse results of energy shortfall in the body. Weight loss through brown fat activity has no rebound effect. In effect, it short-circuits the usual calorie intake/output channels as if body fat had been transported to the brown fat and burnt off. The weight loss can be continuous and is permanent.

Also in Chapter 3 I mentioned the natural opiates connected with food ingestion. These opiates, 50 times more potent than morphine, can make a dramatic contribution to normalizing weight. When ingested food is accompanied by opiate release, they stimulate and precipitate the appetite switch-off mechanism leading to the satiety phenomenon.

These opiates not only come into effect when food is ingested, they also have an action on the appetite regulatory centre in the brain, keeping it at a constant normal level. When the appetite setting is abnormally raised as the result of chronic dieting, these opiates can play a powerful corrective role. They do this by prompt normalization of the appetite demand setting.

Like the brown fat, the opiates produce no rebound effect to decrease their weight-loss potential. On the contrary, as you will see, they produce a different rebound effect which is a direct stimulus to the brown fat.

Once the brown fat cells are activated with food ingestion, the process of weight loss has begun. The first wave of heat loss produced at the beginning of the meal will last till the end of the meal. At the same time, the gut opiates are released and transmit their message to the appetite centre in the brain. The appetite setting is at once lowered to normal. Shortly afterwards, the appetite switch-off mechanism comes into force and inhibits further eating. The total opiate effect is brought about, producing a feeling of physical and emotional satiety.

Following this, there is a rebound action from the total opiate effect. The body temperature is lowered and this, by another circuit, once more stimulates the brown fat, the stimulus this time being the specific sensitivity of the brown fat to a lowered body temperature. The brown fat responds by generating further heat, thus burning off more calories.

The first wave of heat loss starts at the commencement of eating and tails off at the end of the meal. The second wave begins soon afterwards, lasting longer than the first; it can be made to last until the next meal, during which time calories continue to be burnt off.

From the above, you will see that the body has the inherent capacity to normalize its own weight. Briefly, when properly activated, the opiates reduce the appetite setting to its normal level. It then demands only the exact number of calories that the body needs. At the same time, the brown fat is converting calories rapidly into heat and dissipating them. There is net, non-recoverable calorie loss. There is no interference with other bodily systems and functions, which remain normal and unaffected, including those concerned with energy balance.

Both the brown fat and the opiate systems are connected with a rich blood supply. The chemical changes in the blood arising from the activity of these systems act and react in a way which supports the stability of energy balance and all other systems, yet allowing weight to be lost.

By the proper activation of the brown fat and opiate systems, meal after meal of unrestrained eating can be taken. At every meal an increased number of calories will be converted into heat. Further calories will be lost in-between meals via heat formation until the desired weight is attained.

If you wish to accelerate the speed of weight loss, the appetite setting can be lowered 10 per cent below normal. The food intake will then be 10 per cent less than the body's needs. This discrepancy will be absorbed by the greater efficiency of the metabolic processes. It will not cause any resistance, or arouse any defence mechanisms or rebound weight gain.

There is, however, one major obstacle to the recruitment of the brown fat and opiates in the cause of weight loss. These and other weight regulating metabolic processes are all governed by the involuntary nervous system and cannot therefore be controlled by direct conscious effort as such.

There is a way, and a natural way, whereby ordinary voluntary acts can be used in a such a way that they

The two possible outcomes of ingested food in respect of body weight are:

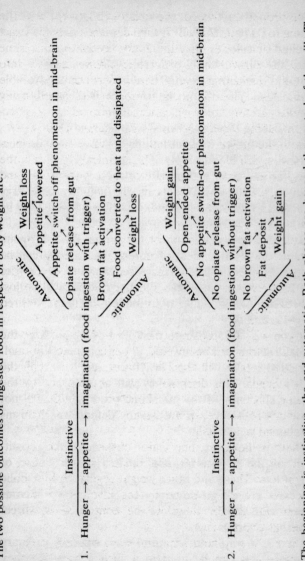

1. Hunger → appetite → imagination (food ingestion with trigger)

   Instinctive

   Automatic
   - Opiate release from gut
   - Appetite switch-off phenomenon in mid-brain
   - Appetite lowered
   - **Weight loss**

   Automatic
   - Brown fat activation
   - Food converted to heat and dissipated
   - **Weight loss**

2. Hunger → appetite → imagination (food ingestion without trigger)

   Instinctive

   Automatic
   - No opiate release from gut
   - No appetite switch-off phenomenon in mid-brain
   - Open-ended appetite
   - **Weight gain**

   Automatic
   - No brown fat activation
   - Fat deposit
   - **Weight gain**

The beginning is instinctive, the end automatic. Both phases are beyond the control of the will. The result is dependent on the presence or absence of the trigger while the food is ingested.

themselves provide links, links which stimulate the involuntary nervous system to act on mechanisms otherwise not under the direct control of the will.

Further, there is a master link which can synchronize, co-ordinate and simultaneously activate all weight regulatory mechanisms otherwise inaccessible to voluntary control.

By a single voluntary act, all weight-control processes and mechanisms can be simultaneously triggered, activated and regulated at will.

In the eating of a meal, the hunger-appetite-imagination-taste components can be normalized by simply removing the restraints on them. Repeated elimination of restraints will automatically revitalize them. But the fact that the food ingested is in keeping with their demands will not in itself activate the weight-reducing phenomena. Only if a link which is under the control of the will is interposed will the systems which will convert food into energy and body fat into heat automatically be activated.

There is only one such trigger, one nervous stimulus, which will automatically activate all the weight-reducing mechanisms simultaneously.

One single use of this trigger can break the vicious circle of weight increase and set it in reverse. The same single application can change the direction of the upward-bound weight-control spiral and reset it in a downward direction. This trigger is the only natural means of weight normalization.

This trigger is the Manorama Formula.

7

The Manorama Formula

The Manorama Formula was born of frustration – impatience with the treatment currently being meted out to the chronically overweight, people who, though clinically healthy, were undergoing unnecessary suffering because of the inadequacies of the 'treatments' then available.

It was evident to me that people with a weight problem followed a universal pattern of weight fluctuation, a see-saw pattern of deliberate weight loss followed by automatic weight regain.

Because I spent part of the year in the West, many people in India consulted me about their weight problems, hoping that I might have a magic recipe for the permanent weight loss which had so far eluded them.

I looked into the existing methods of weight reduction and was not surprised at the almost 100 per cent failure rate. All that was being offered was calorie control either by dieting or by extra exercise, or by a combination of both.

My medical colleagues, both in the West and the East, insisted on calorie control regardless of the fact that their patients returned time after time, still overweight, having regained all the pounds they had so painfully lost.

It was the price in pain these patients paid for their short-lived weight loss that concerned me most. This seemed wrong to me because in nature any procedure which is painful cannot be directed to a positive goal.

I believed that there was real pain in the hunger of starvation. If starvation were not painful, anyone could continue starving indefinitely and so maintain their weight loss. It was equally clear that there was real pain in intensive exercise, because if this were not so anyone could maintain weight loss by continued exhaustive exertion.

I also felt that even if starvation or exercise were the answer to weight problems, nothing so drastic was necessary, because the great majority of people are naturally of normal weight and those who are overweight today were normal in the past. This confirmed that those who were overweight had the capability and the facility to maintain normal weight.

The ability to maintain a steady weight is laid down at birth. There are, however, normal fluctuations in weight. They may be imperceptible but they are always occurring. But though the weight swings back and forth from week to week, from day to day, and even varies during the course of the day, it normally adjusts automatically to its baseline.

When a phase of perceptible weight gain caused by overeating or some other factor is left alone, it will correct itself in the course of time. But if weight loss is enforced by abnormal means, such as starvation or excess exertion, an abnormal element is introduced which sets in motion a chain reaction that defeats the whole purpose.

It was clear to me that this was a short-sighted and illogical approach to the problem, yielding only short-term benefits, achieved at great cost. Artificial interventions prevent the normal corrective mechanism from coming into effect. When they are persisted with over a long period of time, the mechanism for weight adjustment is finally rendered inoperative. A normal situation has been made abnormal.

Clearly this approach was fundamentally erroneous.

I looked at the weight regulatory mechanism in its

totality. I looked at the numerous nervous circuits subscribing to it, the messages they transmitted, and the biochemical changes they produced.

As no one system in the body functions in isolation, I looked at the other systems and their interactions with the weight-control system.

As a specific weight-stabilizing mechanism exists in the body, it was obviously a sound approach to seek to normalize that mechanism rather than to undermine it by introducing abnormal factors. I felt that working with the biological assets of the body instead of against them was the only logical way to solve the hitherto unresolved problem of unstable weight.

The alimentary and nervous systems connected with the ingestion and utilization of food constantly react to each other through a delicate and complex system of checks and balances. If one is checked or controlled on its own, the other reacts in such a way that the overall picture remains unchanged.

You have seen that when food intake is reduced the appetite setting is raised by the nervous system as a compensatory measure to prevent the blood sugar falling to dangerously low levels. The final outcome is that attempts to reduce weight via the alimentary system are rendered futile by the corrective reactions of the nervous system.

I wanted to ensure that the weight-control mechanism was normalized in such a way that the other systems were left undisturbed.

I looked to nature for the answer. The laws of nature are comprehensive and embrace all biological phenomena. Further, nature is the ultimate organizer, co-ordinating collaterally and subordinating hierarchically its many different systems under one unitary law.

I looked to nature because of its consistent tendency to restore normalcy.

Biologically, the nervous system is the primary system governing all the other systems in the body. The human nervous system is the most advanced and sophisticated system in nature. Within this system there are numerous interconnected nervous pathways concerned with weight control. Here again the changes brought about by activating one circuit are balanced by another through biofeedback reactions.

I considered that the only logical approach was through the highest level of control in the brain. By this approach, all the contributory control systems would be automatically normalized. If the problem were tackled through the highest centre in the brain, the balancing reactions that operate when mechanisms at a lower level are interfered with would not arise and the process of weight normalization would proceed in a co-ordinated and physiologically appropriate fashion.

Having decided to approach the issue at the highest level, all that was necessary was to find the right source of natural energy. That energy would be the key factor which would at one stroke resolve the whole issue and normalize the weight-control mechanism at the highest level. It would resolve the entire problem economically and expeditiously.

I also had to make sure that this energy force did not destabilize other systems but worked harmoniously with them. I looked again to nature because nature is not only the ultimate organizer, it is also the ultimate harmonizer. Every system in nature is in harmony with all others.

What I envisaged was something that would at once fulfil all these criteria. However, there was the crucial consideration that most of the bodily functions concerned with weight control are not under the conscious control of the will. Therefore, this energy, if it was to be the key to unlocking the ultimate control mechanism, would in some way have to be brought under the control of the will.

My quest was a simple one because, in the economy of nature, most things are simple. I identified the energy and called it the PP force.

I checked the PP force with the numerous sophisticated systems which make up the weight-control mechanism. I checked it with the different phenomena contained in these systems. I cross-checked it against the fundamental principles of the science of cybernetics (a branch of mathematics applied to the command and control of biological systems). The PP force emerged as the right answer. It had to be right. There is no margin of error in natural phenomena; neither was there in this case.

The PP force is the force of physiological pleasure. Physiological pleasure is not what is usually meant by the term pleasure. It is not limited to the subjective sensations which we recognize as pleasurable. Underlying the subjective sensation of pleasure is a non-subjective component, a system of sensory nerves, sensors, natural opiates and feedback signals. This combination of subjective and non-subjective elements is what is meant by physiological pleasure.

Physiological pleasure is one of the most powerful forms of energy in the body.

Related to the instinct to propagate, physiological pleasure is not only the subjective pleasure of sex, it is that force resulting from the pleasure which brings about the physiological changes in the body which culminate in the fulfilment of the purpose of the instinct – the transmission and implantation of the seed of conception. Physiological pleasure is therefore vital to the creation of life.

In the same way, in relation to the instinct to nourish,

physiological pleasure is crucial for *sustaining* life. Physiological pleasure here is not only the subjective pleasure of eating, it is also that force which brings about the physiological changes which culminate in fulfilling the purpose of eating, i.e. the production of energy and its optimum utilization through maintenance of ideal body weight. Conversely, pleasure ceases when the purpose of eating has been properly fulfilled and further eating is inhibited.

The Manorama Principle as related to biological phenomena asserts that if the phenomenon carries a sensory component, the outcome of the phenomenon will be dependent on the nature of the sensation. If the sensation is pleasurable, it will carry a positive force which will take it towards the desired goal. If the sensation is painful, it will act as a negative force that will move it in the direction opposite to this goal.

As weight reduction by starvation and extra exertion entails pain, the mechanism is forced in an opposite direction to the one desired, by the setting up of double-loop nervous circuits and biofeedback signals operating in the opposite direction. Biologically abnormal methods of weight loss force the control mechanism into the opposite direction from that intended. Further, these nervous impulses are self-perpetuating and have a momentum of their own, a momentum ultimately resulting in a classic example of the vicious circle.

The Manorama Formula is the generation and perpetuation of a force which will be used to break the vicious circle. The continued use of this force will set it in a reverse direction. Once having reversed the spiral, it will automatically generate its own momentum. The initial trigger which sets all these processes in motion is what I named the PP factor.

The PP factor is the direct link between the higher

centres in the brain and the weight-control system in the mid-brain, the link between the conscious voluntary control of the higher centres and the metabolic processes that govern weight control. It is the link which brings these processes under the conscious control of the will.

The PP factor is not something vague and intangible. It is based on well-demarcated anatomical systems of the highest sophistication. It is physiologically precisely defined.

Of the six special senses in the body, taste and smell are importantly involved in food ingestion, sight and the tactile sense also making a major contribution. The only special sense that does not make a contribution to the instinct to nourish is the sense of hearing. The prime importance of the special senses to the instinct to nourish is commensurate with the over-riding importance of nutrition and ideal body build to all other systems.

These are the special senses which initiate physiological pleasure.

Physiological pleasure can be initiated by the interaction of the sensory object, which is food, and the sensory systems of taste and smell at their sites of action. Sensory pleasure is then bonded with the voluntary act of food ingestion. It is perceived in the cortex.

The first interaction of the appropriate food, food in keeping with the demands of hunger and appetite, and the sensory systems initiates a chain reaction in two directions: it stimulates the brown fat and the gut opiate systems in the body. Simultaneously the same interaction is interpreted in the brain and perceived as pleasure. The first interaction in the mouth derives its prime importance from the fact that it facilitates the crucial link, the link between the voluntary act of food ingestion and the recording in the cortex of the brain. The force of physiological pleasure is then transmitted to the weight-control mechanism in the mid-brain. The mid-brain opiates are released and the weight-control mechanism starts to right itself. It also passes on the force to the brown fat and the gut opiate systems and reinforces the activity of these two systems, already activated by the direct act of food ingestion.

Physiological pleasure can not only be precisely defined and qualified, it can be quantified. It can be quantified by the number of cells that are excited and by the intensity with which pleasure is aroused. There are thousands of special cells subscribing to each of the senses, all capable of sending tens of thousands of pleasure signals per minute. The sum total of physiological pleasure will be the combined total of the positive signals sent by the systems involved with the sight, smell, taste and texture of food.

Physiological pleasure can not only be qualified and quantified, it can be multiplied. It cannot be multiplied by direct conscious effort as such. It can be done only by operating the principles of the Manorama Formula.

There is a vast potential for untapped physiological pleasure which can be recruited at will. Further, by eliminating and rejecting food capable of sending negative signals, the total input of the PP factor is maximized.

The speed of weight loss will be in keeping with the force of this pleasure. Any negative force will subtract from its force and consequently from the rate of the loss. The greater the total of positive impulses, the greater the force with which the trigger will propel the weight-control mechanism and the related metabolic processes in the right direction.

This force can be expressed by the following formula:

$$\text{PP force} = \frac{\text{no of sensory cells activated x no of times activated}}{\text{unit of food}}$$

The greater the number of cells activated, the greater the PP force. The greater the number of times the cells are activated by the same unit of food, the greater the physiological pleasure.

The size of the unit or the total quantity of food eaten is irrelevant. It is the ratio between the sensory cell activity generated and the unit of food that is important.

The number of nerve cells activated is proportionate to the intensity of pleasure aroused by the unit of food. If the pleasure is below a certain threshold, no cells will be activated. Every nerve cell is governed by the 'all or nothing' law. When the intensity of a stimulus falls below a certain threshold, the cell is not activated and cannot transmit impulses.

With food ingestion, if insufficient pleasure is generated, the cells will fail to become activated. When the intensity of pleasure meets this threshold the cell is fully activated and cannot be further stimulated for some time by any increase in the intensity of pleasure. The increased intensity is then transmitted by recruiting additional cells which also follow the 'all or nothing' law. Physiological pleasure is then generated by an ever widening circle of cells. The greater the intensity of pleasure, therefore, the greater the number of cells activated.

If the intensity is maintained after the required latency period, the centrally placed cells which were initially stimulated are stimulated once more. Once again, a widening circle of cells is stimulated until eventually all are involved. Therefore, the greater the intensity of the pleasure, the greater the number of times the cells are stimulated per unit of food.

The pleasure of eating is linked with survival. Without pleasure, eating and consequently survival would be in jeopardy. A minimal amount of pleasure is therefore essential for survival.

Reducing diets overrule the pleasure of eating. In chronic dieting, progressively less and less pleasure from eating is generated. When the diet is discontinued, the ability to generate physiological pleasure from eating remains blunted. Disproportionately large amounts of food are required to generate the minimal amount of pleasure that is crucial to survival, resulting in a proportionate reduction in the PP force and consequent reduction in the efficiency of the weight-control processes.

This inefficiency is aggravated by the lack of pleasure through the time factor. Because a minimal amount of pleasure from eating is vital, to obtain this at the earliest opportunity food is eaten at the fastest possible rate. Progressively larger and larger amounts of food are eaten in the shortest possible time to obtain the minimal amount of pleasure necessary for survival. The ratio between quantity of food and pleasure is rendered more abnormal, with a commensurate reduction in the PP force.

Conscious efforts to increase the time taken to consume a unit of food will not correct the equation. By following the Manorama Principle, the number of impulses and the number of times they are transmitted per unit of food will automatically increase to the optimum. The abnormalities of the equation will automatically correct themselves. The formula will then become operative.

The PP factor, as we have seen, consists of two components: firstly, the subjective pleasure which is generated at the site of the sensory systems after they have interacted with external stimuli, and its simultaneous interpretation as pleasure by the brain and secondly, the underlying non-subjective component which is the force transmitted to bring about corresponding physiological changes inside the body.

Spontaneous weight control in a healthy person

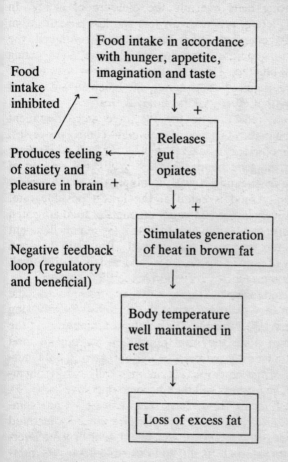

Food intake in accordance with hunger, appetite, imagination and taste

Food intake inhibited −

+ ↓

Releases gut opiates

Produces feeling of satiety and pleasure in brain +

+ ↓

Stimulates generation of heat in brown fat

Negative feedback loop (regulatory and beneficial)

↓

Body temperature well maintained in rest

↓

Loss of excess fat

Regulatory here means that either a transient weight gain or a transient weight loss is brought back to normal. In the language of cybernetics this is a negative feedback loop.

Disruption of weight control through dieting

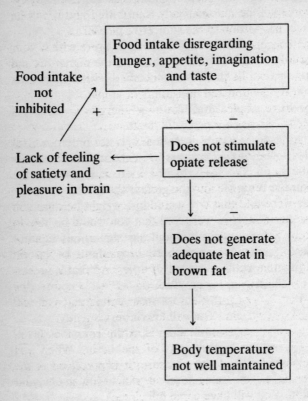

In the language of cybernetics this is a positive feedback loop – a vicious circle of suffering and displeasure is set up, leading to a discontinuation of the diet and a feeling of defeat in the dieter.

You will be concerned only with the subjective element – the generation and promotion of pleasure. The underlying force will be automatically transmitted and it will be in direct proportion to the subjective pleasure.

The trigger which has the power to bring within your control the weight-control mechanism, the numerous and diverse metabolic processes concerned with energy activation, conduction and utilization, is simple.

The force of pleasure, like most energies in nature, is simple to harness but powerful in effect.

When used as nature intended, it is not only powerful but it can be tapped repeatedly without diminishing its resources. On the contrary, the more it is utilized, the quicker the response and the greater the force.

You were told that you would lose weight because you had so decided. You were told that you would be able to do so by natural means, without introducing any unnatural factors, without using harmful methods of calorie manipulation, without the use of drugs. All that is necessary to implement your decision is to generate the maximum amount of pleasure from eating and you will actively lose weight. You will lose it permanently.

The seat of decision-making is at the conscious level, which is in the highest part of the brain. When you consciously acknowledge pleasure, it is perceived at the highest level, the same level at which you made your decision. You will have come full circle.

You will be concerned with the generation of pleasure at the initial site of food intake and the perception and conscious acknowledgement of pleasure at the highest level of the brain. Both are under the control of the will. Between these two sites you will then set up a direct master nervous circuit which becomes operative immediately. Via feedback systems it will become self-perpetuating. These activities at these two sites can be activated consciously whenever you wish, thereby bringing the master pathway under your control. This circuit is an additional direct and independent one which circumvents and overrides the direct pathways to the gut opiates and the brown fat in the body.

The perception of pleasure generates a force which acts on the weight-control mechanism at a lower level in the mid-brain, which is otherwise not under the direct control of the will. The weight-control mechanism, when activated, will in turn influence the lower-level nervous centres and the metabolic processes. Thus the main route for normalizing the weight-control mechanism stems directly from pleasure via the highest centre of the brain and passes down the central nervous system. This is the central, primary, powerful channel of force that will implement your decision to lose weight. This is the route which will correct the central weight-control mechanism.

In the last chapter you saw how the same trigger, i.e. physiological pleasure, will bring about weight loss through the direct and visceral channel. You saw that when you allowed free rein to the natural flow of the hunger-appetite-imagination sequence, and linked the trigger of pleasure to the voluntary act of eating, it led through the peripheral channels to the activation of the gut opiate systems and the brown fat.

The opiates normalize the appetite and the brown fat causes weight loss.

You have seen that these activities work individually towards the common goal of weight normalization. You have seen that there is, in addition, an interplay of the two systems which compounds and accelerates weight loss. At the onset of food ingestion, when that food produces pleasure, the excitatory nervous system is activated, and this in turn stimulates brown fat activity. This generates heat, the dissipation of which causes weight loss. Also, at the onset of a meal which generates physiological pleasure, the opiate system starts releasing opiates. When a sufficient number have been released to satisfy the hunger-appetite criterion, they operate the switch-off mechanism in the mid-brain and the total satiety effect which precludes further eating comes into being. This effect, which affects the total being at all levels, physical, emotional and intellectual, is so completely satisfactory that to maintain the status quo further eating becomes undesirable.

As you have seen, the rebound action of the opiate effect lowers the body temperature which in turn activates the brown fat through its thermogenic stimulus. The second activity, though mediated through a different nervous circuit, arises from the same trigger. For the second time, wave after wave of heat is produced and lost. It is lost because the body temperature does not need to be raised and the heat generated is superfluous. This wave of weight loss is longer than the first, which is limited to the time at which the food is ingested. It can last till the next cycle of hunger demanding food intake arises. An organized and continuous process of weight loss is set in motion.

The intellectual or mental force from the highest centre in the brain travels down to the mid-brain weight-control mechanism, which reacts automatically according to the principles of cybernetics. It 'commands and controls'. It orders the body fat cells to release fat into the blood-stream. It orders the brain fat cells to lower it.

This is the route which will be responsible for permanent weight control.

This single trigger, i.e. perception of pleasure, simultaneously and harmoniously activates two channels, bringing the mental, sensory and involuntary activities and energies towards the common goal of weight loss at all levels.

The time factor is a crucial element in the equation. When abnormally large quantities of food are eaten in less than the metabolically optimal time, the PP force is diminished. This cannot be corrected by slower eating. Correction will come about automatically when the PP force is generated with regularity and with maximum intensity, i.e. when the maximum pleasure over a maximum period of time is obtained per unit of food. When this ratio is achieved, it is an indication that the internal mechanism has corrected itself.

Preferred food in preferred quantities at preferred times lays down the foundation of weight regulation. When you eat what you want, as much as you want, when you want, you have the best chance of generating and perceiving pleasure. Once having relearnt to generate and perceive pleasure from your food, even meals of second choice will evoke it. You will be able to derive physiological pleasure and its benefits even when food of your first choice is not available. Third world communities, which are invariably denied choice, use the PP factor to great advantage. They fulfil the primary purpose of eating against heavy odds.

More importantly, once having regenerated the central weight-control mechanism itself, if for some reason you are not eating your preferred food, the revitalized weight-stabilizing mechanism will maintain a stable weight despite any excess eating which may have come about by the non-availability of first-choice food or for any other reason. You will not have to concern yourself with the brown fat activity and the opiate release. They will be operating automatically whenever you ingest food when you follow the Manorama Formula. You will only be concerned with the master circuit.

You will recall that I proposed bringing all the phenomena under voluntary control through a common link, a single link which would be interposed between the voluntary act of food ingestion and between all the involuntary phenomena leading to weight loss and control.

That single crucial link is not at the site of the first interaction between sensory systems in the mouth and the sense objects, which is a mechanical interaction only. The determining link is the link between food ingestion and the primary weight-control mechanism in the midbrain. The link is made in the cortex in the highest part of the brain. It is in the cortex that the perception of physiological pleasure is seated. You will be concerned with this perception and nothing else.

The weight control mechanism is not under the control of the intelligence or the will. It is part of the vegetative or instinctive systems we possess in common with the lower animals. But it can be brought under the control of the will by one force only, the force of pleasure perceived in the cortex. This perception is the total Manorama Formula.

When food is ingested, the perception of pleasure from the taste buds acts as a stimulus which reinforces the brown fat activity. It also acts as a stimulus to the gut opiates which reinforce the action of the mid-brain opiates acting on the weight-control mechanism, which further rights itself. The whole weight-regulation process is set up in an organized and cohesive way to lead to weight loss.

You have seen that for practical purposes the Manorama Formula has been reduced for you to one single operation – i.e., the perception of pleasure. The Manorama Formula can make the brain and the entire nervous system work mechanically and automatically to achieve weight control permanently.

The brain can be made to work as a combination of mechanical devices operated by the stimulus of pleasure.

To lose and stabilize weight, one stimulus will activate various mechanical devices in the brain in appropriate sequence. Once activated, the message is transmitted unchanged, electromechanically via the nerves, to the energy-regulating systems which adjust mechanically and automatically.

To lose weight by activation of the opiate systems and the brown fat, the stimulus of anticipated pleasure switches on a mechanical device in the brain whereby hunger, appetite and choice of food are computed with absolute precision.

Pleasure associated with eating is firstly transmitted electromechanically, instantaneously and without change, by the nerves to the cortex, from whence it is transmitted downwards to the mid-brain weight-control system, which reacts immediately and mechanically and initiates the process of immediate weight loss. Secondly, having been transmitted, the experience is not erased from the cortex but is codified and banked for further reference. This establishes the basis for permanent weight loss.

Further similar pleasurable experiences reinforce the memory. In due course, progressively strong and clear messages are codified and stored. The brain has then become programmed.

A computer works in an exactly similar way. When one key is pressed, a particular message is transmitted mechanically, unchanged. Only one particular programme is then decodified. The same programme is retrieved on cue every time that key is pressed.

In weight regulation, perception of pleasure associated with food is the key. When pressed, only one particular message can be transmitted – the message to redress weight imbalance and to maintain ideal body weight. The same response will be produced on cue every time you eat, because the cortex will have been programmed to respond to the stimulus of food ingestion in one specific way. Once pleasure is perceived, the entire weight-loss process, including the recording and programming, become mechanical. Even on occasions when food is ingested without positive identification of pleasure, the programmed cortex will continue to send appropriate messages.

One of the consequences of perceived pleasure is the unique result of *maintaining* weight loss. There is no other tenable substitute which will maintain it. Though weight loss is possible by other means, unacceptable though they may be, there is no other way, acceptable or unacceptable, which will retain the lost weight except the Manorama Formula.

The programme from perceived pleasure to ideal weight is laid down at birth. Every normal child is born with a unique build of exquisite proportions. Western communities, more so than in the less affluent East, are subject to enormous commercial pressures which conflict with the inner signals and reduce pleasure. Deprived of the stimulus of pleasure, the programme in the cortex is depleted and becomes ineffective. Without nervous input from the computer, the weight-control mechanism lower down in the mid-brain becomes rudderless. It then becomes governed by the secondary channels which react primarily to the blood sugar level, a level which is lowered by the insufficient calories of reducing diets, raising the appetite and resulting in rebound weight regain.

The pleasure of eating is linked with survival. Therefore, most people who eat without dietary restriction perceive pleasure to a reasonable degree. They therefore achieve a reasonable degree of weight control and a reasonable energy flow instinctively. When you consciously recharge the programme, you become the programmer. You will have 100 per cent control. You will have the perfect body weight and proportions you had at birth.

The perception of pleasure is the beginning and the end.

8
Practical application

Pleasure, the basis of your weight-control formula, is a powerful biological stimulus. It is also the most powerful natural incentive to your goal. It will revitalize your whole energy system. It will redress your weight imbalance.

You already possess the machinery for controlling your weight. You have a healthy hunger, appetite, imagination and sense of taste. You are now aware of their value and significance and of how you can properly use them both for immediate pleasure and for long-term goal fulfilment.

You have looked at the body as a whole and into the mechanics of the weight-regulation processes. You have seen their interaction with related systems. You have taken into account the factor of individual variations. You know the significance of the body's energy systems and the vitalizing role they play in all the activities of life. You now have sufficient information to achieve your goal, information based on the most comprehensive scientific data, yet which has been simplified for you. You are now equipped to implement your decision to lose weight. You are now independent of every restraint. You are free to regain control over yourself.

To derive the maximum benefit from your own natural endowments of hunger and appetite, all you need now do is to disregard obsolete preconceptions. Guilt in the pleasure of eating is not only counterproductive, in biological terms it is entirely misplaced. As we have seen, pleasure is the ultimate criterion by which the body measures its nutritional needs and the final instrument in correcting faulty eating. As survival is dependent on eating, the accompanying pleasure is entirely legitimate. There is no factor which can mitigate the total legitimacy of pleasure.

Reducing diets make a virtue of the pain of starvation. By implication, the pleasure of eating is made out to be something which is in some way unacceptable and therefore to be discouraged. This can induce powerful feelings of guilt associated with eating, negative feelings which have no place in nature's scheme of energy incrementation. Neither have they any place in the Manorama Formula. In nature, eating is a total self-enhancing phenomenon. You will find it will be so for you.

Initially, the Manorama Formula requires a small investment in time. This will, however, be for a short and temporary period only. You will not only quickly recover your investment, you will have regularly accruing dividends for all time. You will have abundant energy, not only for voluntary muscular activity, but also for the optimal functioning of all the involuntary systems of the body. You will have weight stabilization throughout your life.

Guilt in spending time in eating is as equally misplaced as guilt in gaining pleasure from eating. The French as a nation probably devote more time to the preparation and enjoyment of food than any other race. With their sophisticated culinary skills, the time and care they give to the selection, preparation and cooking of food, even the time they spend talking about it, they have raised the enjoyment derived from food to a fine art. They extract the maximum amount of pleasure not only from the eating of their meals but from the anticipatory enjoyment derived from planning and cooking them. All this is life-enhancing in itself, but it has the additional bonus of producing a super-efficient metabolism which provides ample ready energy and speedily burns up any excess calories they may ingest. Thus, in spite of their enjoyment and interest in food, the French as a nation have no difficulty in maintaining reasonable and stable levels of weight.

Unrestrained choice is pleasure-producing. To give full expression to your choice, and above all to vary it when you so desire, is pleasure-enhancing. The more food options you have, the greater the opportunity for pleasure and the greater your personal fulfilment and individual development.

Choice of food is an individual affair. Two members of the same family may have totally different food preferences. Your individual food preferences reflect your body's needs and your individuality.

When I first introduce overweight people to the principles of the Manorama Formula, almost without exception they express doubts about this single factor. They believe that taking pleasure in eating will lead automatically to overeating. In fact, overeating is the direct result, not of too much pleasure in eating, but of too little. Sufficient pleasure from eating inhibits overeating.

Another area of concern many people have is that by freely giving in to their individual food preferences they will automatically eat more and more of one particular food. A common fear of those who like sweets or chocolates, for instance, is that they will eat chocolate and little else, which would be harmful. There are no grounds for anxiety on this account. With any individual food preference, there is a clear cut-off point when its usefulness to the body is fulfilled. Pleasure from the food in question will then cease and there will be a natural disinclination to eat further. When the systems are functioning correctly, there is a built-in switch-off mechanism which comes into effect when enough of *any* particular food has been eaten. Eating beyond that point causes revulsion.

By restricting the choice of food, diets not only create an insufficiency of pleasure, they also lay down the chemical basis of food addiction. The body reacts to its unfulfilled needs by continuing to transmit signals until food occupies every area of the dieter's thoughts.

You are now familiar with the principles of the Manorama Formula. All that remains for you to do now is to apply them. It is a simple process.

At some time or another you will, in practice, have applied the principles of the Manorama Formula. You will have eaten a valued meal in your favourite surroundings in a restaurant of your choice, and you will have devoted your time and attention exclusively to your meal. You will have chosen from the menu exactly what gave you most pleasure at the time. You will have gained a full measure of satisfaction from the comfort of your surroundings, from making your choice from the menu, and from the pleasure of anticipating your favourite dishes. You will have savoured the aroma and viewed the attractively served food with appreciation. With appetite and hunger now at their peak, you will have eaten the food with the maximum amount of pleasure, giving it your full attention and a generous measure of your time. Finally, at the end of your meal, you will have experienced the satiety phenomenon of overwhelming benefit to body and mind.

This could become your model, a model you can reproduce in your own home at every meal with only a little initial organization.

The first essential in preparing your model meal is freedom of choice. Choice based on personal preference rather than on any outside dictates should be the first criterion of the selection of your menu. Your food preferences will vary constantly according to the changing needs of your body. To give them free rein, keep in stock a wide variety of the ingredients of your favourite dishes. Within your resources, have a ready supply of these foods to hand. Only when you are equipped to fulfil last-minute changes in your preferences will you have total choice.

Desire for a particular item of food arising at a particular time has a valid physiological basis. The body's needs are constantly changing and this is reflected in the arousal of a desire for a particular food at a particular time. A good example of the perfect matching of the body's needs to the appearance of a strong desire for a particular food is in pregnancy, when the nutritional demands on the mother are considerable and are moreover rapidly changing, and the craving for some particular food item suddenly arises. That food item will contain a nutrient that has become exhausted and the body is signalling the need for speedy replenishment.

The presentation of food makes an important contribution to the pleasure of eating. It is important because the sight of a well-prepared dish, cooked in the way you most prefer, and attractively presented, is the first pleasure stimulus. The smell of your favourite flavours is the accompanying pleasure stimulus.

Flavourings of your choice contribute to the pleasure obtained from a well-prepared meal and should be chosen with care and discrimination. Almost all reducing diets eliminate or drastically reduce salt, sugar and butter, condiments which contribute to making food appetizing and palatable. As we have seen, all these foods are health-inducing and non-fattening. Their palatability value is based on sound biological considerations. They reflect the body's nutritional needs and to eliminate them is to reject these needs. Unflavoured meats, vegetables eaten raw and without condiments, and insipid salads, the staple foods of reducing diets, deprive you of the pleasure of eating for no biologically valid reason.

Food addiction resulting from chronic dieting instils an element of urgency if food is not readily available. So compulsive can this addiction become that some dieters can hardly wait to take food from its carton; they will eat the food which is most readily to hand, even eating food directly from the refrigerator, or gulping down foods normally disliked to satisfy their craving for the act of eating. The ready availability of a favourite meal will counteract panic eating. In due course the experience of readily available satisfactory meals will eradicate it altogether. You will be in control of your meals and will therefore have a positive feeling of overall control.

So organize your meal in anticipation of the hunger which must inevitably arise, so that the demands of hunger-appetite-taste do not have to wait for the meal; rather the meal which will meet their demands in every detail will await the call of your inner signals.

External signals from the environment should be such that they enhance the pleasure from your meal. Any negative signal – noise, cold, or constant interruptions – will detract from the total pleasure of your meal. Create a pleasant environment for eating and eliminate all sources of unpleasant or irritating stimuli.

Neutralize any painful or uncomfortable personal stimuli. Comfortable seating arrangements will contribute to your total comfort and relaxation.

When your body is relaxed and comfortable and your surroundings are harmonious, your mind will be free to focus on the pleasure you gain from your meal.

When you are ready to eat, when all your external and internal signals are positive ones of comfort and pleasure, and your inner signals tell you that hunger and appetite are at their peak, identify the pleasure from the sight and aroma of your food. Choose your additional flavourings with deliberation and care. Serve yourself generous helpings.

Generous helpings will not make you overeat. Many people who consult me about their weight problems at first find this difficult to accept. I explain to them that the body regulates its appetite according to its needs rather than according to the availability of the food; scarcity of food, or even the thought of scarcity, increases the body's demands as a safeguard against future deprivation. With experience, these people gradually come to realize that they are, in fact, actually eating less than they had previously. They are burning their calories instead of conserving them against future scarcity. Once they have given up even the thought of limiting their food intake, all the rest falls into place.

The size and number of helpings, the size of individual mouthfuls, are irrelevant in themselves. What is relevant is the amount of pleasure they contribute. This is a personal variable. Only you can decide the quantity that will give you the most pleasure. The essential thing is that you identify the quantity and derive the greatest possible pleasure from that unit which is your preferred measure.

When you have had a sufficient sum total of pleasure from the planning and sight, smell, taste and texture of food, you will automatically achieve satiety.

Recognize the satiety experience at its onset. Note the physical, emotional and mental satisfaction. You will have a natural, recognizable, and strong disinclination to eat further. Overruling this inclination is wasteful. Your body has signalled that it does not require any more food. Finishing what is left on your plate is not eliminating waste, it is wasteful in itself. The extra food will not produce extra energy. Ceasing to eat beyond the point of satiety will in due course enable you to estimate your portions exactly. Waste will then be truly eliminated.

Note the comfort of a full stomach. The stretch reflexes in the stomach and their subsidiary feedback loops are the primary systems which check food intake for bulk. For the efficient functioning of the entire digestive system there is an optimal bulk. Too little or too much bulk detracts from this efficiency. Appetite and taste not only regulate food intake for its nutritional value, they also regulate it for its bulk factor. This is then double-checked by the stomach. For example, a shortage of vitamin C may need two or three oranges to correct it. The appetite will not only make the correction in respect of the 200 to 300 calories involved, it will adjust the correction in respect of their bulk value also. If the same deficiency is fulfilled by, say, lemon juice, then the appetite will not only take into account the lower number of calories involved but the lesser bulk as well, and will come to the precise equation of bulk requirement in both cases. There is no other known system in existence able to make this computation. On it depends the health of the whole gastrointestinal tract, and external dictates can never match its precision.

Bran is promoted for its bulk value. But as it has no nutritional value, you automatically eat more to compensate for the lack. This causes overstretch, which is counter-productive and harmful. The system reacts by rapid movement to reject the superfluous and harmful substance. In so doing, the absorption of the remainder of the food is interfered with. In fact, bran disturbs the stomach's bulk-computing mechanism to the detriment of the overall metabolic processes. In time it weakens it and renders it defective.

Diets have no provision for individual bulk requirements or for the personal status of the gastrointestinal
tract. They therefore cause overstretch or understretch
of the whole tract from the stomach downwards, with
consequent disturbance of function. In due course, after
a period of instinctive eating, you will be able to estimate
the exact amount of food from which the stomach will be
neither understretched nor overstretched. Though the
stretch signals emit from the stomach only, the stomach
estimates the optimal bulk for the whole of the gastrointestinal system, that bulk which is conducive to the
maintenance of a good physical state and efficient functioning. If any damage has already occurred, it will be
rectified.

While you are gaining pleasure from your meal, you
must consciously recognize and acknowledge this pleasure. In this way, the fact will be recorded in your brain.
When you have consciously recorded pleasure from a
sufficient number of meals, your brain will have become
programmed to react automatically to every meal with
a release of opiates and the stimulation of brown fat
activity.

Initially you may feel that this will take up more time
than you can spare for yourself. But whatever the time
spent on creating a model meal, regard it as rightfully
yours as a priority, a priority taking precedence over any
other need.

Many people who consult me about their weight problems initially demur at the extra expenditure of time.
Much of their hesitation arises from feelings of guilt over
spending time on themselves rather than from any actual
shortage of time. However, they soon come to realize
that the extra time spent on preparing and eating their
model meal is productive in time as well as in health and
well-being. With their increased energy, they actually

increase the time they have to spare for their other interests. In due course, they find also that they are spending less time in creating their model meal because the guidelines are already there. They become more and more easy to put into effect.

Another area of concern to many of my overweights was their feelings of lack of control. They felt that they would not be able to control nibbling or eating between meals, or eating what they considered harmful foods such as sweets, chocolates or savoury snacks. My advice was not to force any changes, but in fact to allow themselves the maximum number of options. Craving for sweets and snacks between meals arises because of an insufficient release of opiates during the meal, giving rise to nagging, unsatisfied desires leading to constant nibbling. Restraints were entirely counter-productive. As soon as they had learnt to derive complete satisfaction from the meals themselves, they ceased to nibble. The total freedom from anxiety about food in-between meals and the time it saved them was a priceless reward.

These then are your guidelines. From the beginning to the end, you have only one aim, that of the conscious perception of pleasure. You have no other target. Hunger, appetite, imagination, the sense of taste, can all have a righting effect on weight regulation. But in the last analysis they are all overchecked by pleasure – pleasure you need to sustain, acknowledge and record.

9
How to manipulate your signals

You now know in detail the signals which lead to the pleasure of eating and those painful signals which detract from the sum total of that pleasure.

You have your general guidelines as to how to recruit positive signals and eliminate negative signals.

The inner signals related to the instinct of eating are always present. Regardless of how much they are misused, disused or abused, they can be revitalized. Once they are strengthened, they can be easily recorded and interpreted. It will then be possible to respond to them effectively.

The rehabilitation of the weight-control mechanism is expedited by expedient recovery of strong inner signals. Identifiable signals, uninhibited by conflicting messages, further speed the recovery of the weight-control mechanism.

Once you have regained recognition of your signals and familiarized yourself with them, you will have initiated the weight-regulating process. As you have seen, the rest is instinctive. It leads to a natural progression culminating in pleasure.

If you are able to reproduce and promote your positive inner signals at will and eliminate your negative signals you will then have gained real control.

The three specific positive signals are feelings of satiety, of fullness of the stomach, and of general warmth and well-being. The two specific negative signals are feelings of tension or discomfort from either internal or external parts of the body.

Just as you have seen that the brain can be made to work chemico-mechanically and naturally, you will now be shown that you can also generate positive signals and eliminate negative signals chemico-mechanically by means of certain natural food substances.

There are certain valuable natural substances of exceptional quality which you can use specifically to highlight your positive signals or to abolish each and every negative signal. Through the use of these substances you can target them with precision. They have been used in the East for centuries, not only to highlight or abolish inner signals, but to rejuvenate, recharge and exploit the entire energy system. They can be used to manipulate all the above-mentioned five signals.

1) *Jas*. This is a preparation made out of extracts of various plants of one parent family, one of the ingredients being the extract of the plant *ephedra*. It has been used in India for centuries. For the last 100 years, the alkaloid of *ephedra* has also been used in Western medicine for a variety of conditions because it is a sympatheticomimetic activator, that is, it mimics the action of the sympathetic nervous system. Jas lowers the appetite setting and satisfies the appetite component of the weight-reduction mechanism. By using this at your convenience you will be able to identify and alter your appetite setting. You will become familiar with appetite satisfaction. As it happens, this substance, by means of its sympatheticomimetic action, simultaneously activates the brown fat, bringing about feelings of warmth which you will learn to recognize. Through its use you will have begun the process of weight loss.

Though I have been using the plant extract for some time, researchers at Cambridge University and other institutions have recently started experimenting with excellent results with a laboratory-produced substance identical in chemical composition for the purpose of activating brown fat. I anticipate that this will be taken up by commercial interests and hailed as a breakthrough. But I believe that the introduction of this substance for weight-loss purposes will cause the same problems as weight loss by dieting. As soon as use of the substance is discontinued, the weight will be regained. Its use by-passes the factor of pleasure from the ingestion of food, which is the only natural, permanent way of weight control. It will be a temporary help only, because the causes of brown fat degeneration will have remained uncorrected. In the Manorama Formula, the pleasure evoked at every meal is the only complete answer. I anticipate that in due course the status of this substance in weight-control regimes will decline to that of a limited-value substance only, as happened to the chemical appetite suppressants which at one time were hailed as a breakthrough.

However, in the short term, Jas has a valid place in the identification, regeneration and recharging of your signals at will, and in starting you off on your weight-loss programme. But it does not have a permanent place in weight reduction independent of the principles of the Manorama Formula.

In the short term it will help to identify the feeling of all-over warmth consequent on its activation of the brown fat, and can be used for this whenever you wish. Once you have learnt to recognize this feeling you will readily identify its arousal after a pleasurable meal, when it will confirm the fact that your meal has succeeded in converting you into a fast burner.

2) *Ram*. Made from a special soft variety of plant seed grown in certain areas of India with a cold dry climate,

mostly in wild inaccessible regions of the country. Its main ingredient is 'fleaseed', together with other seeds of the same family. Ram is an efficient and effective natural filler, or bulking agent, perhaps the only known filler in nature. No other food or plant substance is as effective for this purpose. Attempts at making artificial fillers have failed up to now. You will at once be able to see its action for yourself – a large spoonful of this food, made up in a cup of milk or water, will form a semi-solid gelatinous mass ten times its original bulk. It is this consistency that gives it its special quality of arousing feelings of fullness in the stomach, which you have seen has an important role in appetite control and efficient functioning of the gastrointestinal tract. With the help of this substance you will be able to generate at will and identify this fullness. After you have done so a few times you will be able to anticipate fullness of the stomach at your meals and will not overeat.

3) *Prith*. A berry mixed with a small but specific proportion of herbs in syrup. Its main ingredient is *embelic myrobalam*. Of all natural substances it has the highest vitamin C content. It thus has a high biological value far and above any other natural or synthetic source of the vitamin. A recent investigation undertaken by the Asian Congress of Pharmacology at New Delhi showed that in a group of people given 100 mg of synthetic vitamin C their blood level of the vitamin was raised by 110.065 per cent after one day; in another group given the vitamin in its natural form it was raised by 973 per cent; whereas when Prith was given to the third group the level rose by 1156.48 per cent. Moreover, the berry, which is the main ingredient of Prith, is the only source of vitamin C in which the full vitamin content is retained even when it is dried and powdered.

But Prith derives its special importance from the fact that it contains a chemical substance which is identical to metabolized food in its penultimate cycle, before it converts to energy in the form of blood sugar. Within minutes of taking it you will find that you will have abundant physical energy. You can take it at any time to become familiar with the component of the satiety phenomenon which ensues after hunger is satisfied and ready energy becomes available. With this syrup you can generate this energy and satiety feeling at will at any time.

4) *Pra*. An aromatic compound of natural herbs which has a high potency for neutralizing tension, pain and discomfort. Its main ingredients are menthol, thymol and eucalyptus oil. Its tincture form ensures its prompt absorption into the bloodstream and immediate circulation to all parts of the body, producing prompt relief of symptoms. About 10 drops in half a cup of water will neutralize internal pain or discomfort in any part of the body and specifically in the alimentary tract. Any internal pain, discomfort or unease will perforce distract from the total pleasure of eating. You can use this substance at will to eliminate any negative signals that may be present and to relax and ease the internal system to maximize the pleasure of your meal.

5) *Tab*. A compound of natural herbs for external use with a high potency for neutralizing pain or discomfort, or any unease of joints or muscles. It is an oily substance consisting of methyl salicilate, eucalyptus oil, pumilio oil and menthol which when used on the skin is spontaneously absorbed. Here again its use is primarily to eliminate at will any distractions from the pleasure of eating coming from negative signals from the exterior of the body.

In the East all these substances are available across the counter from herbalists. Not all Western herbalists stock them, but they are available from Shree BCM Shree Sharan, London WC1N 3XX.

Through the use of these foods and herbs and their chemicomechanical action you can eliminate the two groups of negative signals at will and generate each and every one of the three positive signals related to food ingestion. You will gain control over your pleasure-generating signals.

All these substances potentiate pleasure and promote comfort and ease. With a little experience you can use them at any convenient time, and they will expeditiously prepare you for the rectification of your weight-control mechanism.

By making it possible for you to generate feelings of satiety, fullness of stomach and general warmth at will, by enabling you to eliminate any external or internal tension and discomfort at will, these small but valuable herbs and foods are useful for attaining mastery over your signals; that is their only purpose. It is incidental that while you are familiarizing yourself with the Manorama Formula, weight loss will have been initiated.

Once you have learnt the Formula, with or without the assistance of these substances, you will be in complete control of your weight and you should discontinue their use; they will have served their purpose. If in the future you should wish to manipulate any one of your five signals, you can make selective use of them for this purpose.

10
Success guaranteed – case histories

Introducing my patients to the Manorama system was a rewarding experience. Many of them had undergone years of deprivation. Some had run the entire gamut of diets, clinics and health farms without success. They now found themselves free to eat when and what they liked for the first time in years.

At first they found it difficult to believe that a regime which did not involve diet or exercise could really reduce their weight, but as they gained confidence they found that this was indeed so. The system worked in every case. These patients' weight has remained stable over the years and they have been liberated from the long years of deprivation and self-sacrifice. A few individual case histories illustrate how the system worked in different patients.

Mr K was a contracting engineer. He had been of normal weight all his life, weighing 12 stone at the age of 34, a normal weight for his height of 6 feet. At this stage he began working on building a satellite township outside Delhi, and had to live on the site for three months at a time, leaving his family behind in the city. On the construction site, life was fairly primitive and he lived in a hut with one servant to cater for his needs and cook his meals. The meals were less palatable than he was used to and he began to eat more to relieve the unsatisfied feelings the food produced. During the evenings he was alone and began to drink more to relieve his loneliness. He started putting on weight and because there was a family history of hypertension, he was urged to go on a diet. From then on his life followed the familiar pattern of diet/weight loss/normal eating/weight regain. He augmented the diet with exercise, performing 100 press-ups a day, all to no avail.

When I saw him three years later he was 15 stone, three stone above his original weight. I recognized his problem immediately. During his tours away from home he had paid scant attention to his food, eating everything his servant provided and augmenting this with a fairly large alcohol intake. At home on leave, with palatable, well-prepared meals, he had not gained weight and in due course his weight would probably have reverted to its original level, but by going on a reducing diet he had set in motion the inevitable progression towards obesity that comes from dieting, with inhibition of the brown fat activity and slowing of the body's metabolic rate.

Mr K's wife had brought him to see me hoping I would be able to supply some new miracle diet from the West. At first they found it hard to accept that no dieting was involved. But once initiated, Mr K immediately began a steady weight loss. When I saw him again seven or eight months later he had lost the three stone he had accumulated. He is still at a stable weight after seven years.

As a child, **CJ** had been of normal weight. Both her parents were slim and ate whatever they liked without weight gain. At the age of 14, however, CJ's weight started to rise, and at 16 she weighed 11 stone, which for her height of 5′ 2″ was greatly overweight. She was now approaching the time when her parents had to think about arranging her betrothal, and it was feared that her obesity would seriously affect her prospects in the marriage market. So they took her to a homoeopathic doctor who prescribed a diet and gave her a course of appetite suppressants. All her meals were closely supervised by her parents, and in view of the anxiety about her marriage prospects these became charged with tension. By the time I saw her when she was 18 or 19 years old, she had run the entire gamut of one semi-starvation diet after another and was still very fat. She and her parents were at first highly sceptical about my method. But they had tried everything without success and felt that there was nothing to lose by trying it.

I told her parents to stop supervising CJ's meals and to let her eat whatever she wanted. This included items like chocolates and ice cream, which she had not touched for years. But she lost weight, coming down to a normal 8½ to 9 stones in a few months. Moreover, she stayed at that weight. She married at the age of 20 and had two children. After each pregnancy she regained her normal weight without difficulty. She is now in her late 20s and her weight has been stable for years.

Mrs L had been a tall, slender, elegant and attractive woman, moving in the sophisticated jet-setting society of Delhi. She had married young and was now in her early 40s, with her family grown-up and married. Mrs L had always spent a great deal of time and money on her dress and appearance and was proud of her svelte figure. She was scornful of women who 'let themselves go'. But after a traumatic family dispute which resulted in her sons and daughters-in-law leaving home, she put on 20 pounds in weight. This was not a large gain and it certainly did not make her obese, but because of her love of fashionable clothes, and with her adherence to the fashionable figure ideal, she was determined to shed the unwanted pounds as quickly as possible. So she went to a yoga ashram in the mountains and underwent a strict regime of rising at 5.00 A.M. and undergoing a vigorous routine of strenuous

yoga exercises and eating the sparse meals provided by
the institute, where austere living was held to be a virtue.
At the ashram Mrs L certainly lost weight, but she
regained it promptly on her return. She spent further
periods at the ashram but the end result was a weight
gain far in excess of the original 20 pounds she had set
out to lose. She began to take appetite suppressants, but
on these she developed a rapid heart rate and her doctor
advised her to stop them. She began to take the appetite
suppressants clandestinely without her husband's knowledge and despite her doctor's warning. At this stage, in
despair, she finally consulted me. Mrs L soon regained
her original slender figure and was able once more to
indulge her love of fashion. Her weight, too, has remained
stable since then.

Miss H was a successful fashion model, a slender 8½
stone for her height of 5' 8". But at the age of 26 she
sustained a compound fracture of one of her legs and was
immobilized for 10 weeks, during which time she lay
around all day eating chocolates and reading. By the time
her leg was out of plaster, her weight had gone up to 10
stone. As her livelihood depended on her slender figure,
she went on a rigid diet, which succeeded in bringing her
weight down. But any break in the diet resulted in a
massive rebound weight gain – at weekends she would
put on a pound a day, so that a three-day weekend would
result in a weight gain of three pounds. On a two-week
holiday she put on a whole stone. By this time her dieting
was interfering badly with her social life, and from being
an outgoing, sociable girl she became practically a recluse.
In the end, in spite of all her efforts, she was unable to
keep her weight in the fashionable slender mould and
had to give up modelling. When I saw her she had
practically given up the struggle. On the Manorama

Formula she rapidly returned to her normal weight of 8½ stone and was able to resume her modelling career. At the age of 32, she married and had two children with no resulting weight gain. She is still the same weight seven years later.

Miss S was an 18-year-old university student and weighed 9 stone. Her height was 5′ 6″. For some reason she had decided that she wished to be slimmer still and began a rigid diet. She shed a stone in weight on this diet but lost her former good looks, becoming haggard and drawn, with deep circles around her eyes. She became tense, irritable and hyper-excitable. When this had continued for six months her family were reaching the limits of their patience, and her bad temper was beginning to have a bad effect on the whole household. By this time her preoccupation with her weight was becoming obsessive, and in addition to rigid dieting Miss S was also attending a gymnasium where she carried out high-intensity exercising, continuing the programme in her own room in-between her attendances.

When I saw Miss S a year later, she had become completely obsessed with her weight, but at the insistence of her family reluctantly agreed to try the Manorama Formula. Against my advice she was continuing to exercise in secret. However, the friend who had originally brought her to see me was eventually able to persuade her that the Formula would not work for her if she continued to exercise and she gave it up, though with many initial misgivings. To her surprise she found that the Formula did indeed work, without diet and without exercise. She achieved perfect weight control effortlessly and began to lose her obsession with her weight and to enjoy life once more. She regained her former good looks and happy disposition to the great delight of her family, and moreover was full of health and energy. When I saw her a couple of years later, she told me of her enormous relief at having got 'the weight monkey off my back'. She is still the same weight ten years later.

A designer of children's clothes, **Mrs J**, married with two children, had her own business, which she had developed from her hobby of making her own children's clothes. At the age of 32 she weighed about 8½ stone for a height of 5' 5". About four years before I saw her, her husband had had an affair with another woman. The stress of this caused her to seek comfort in eating, and she was soon eating huge quantities of food. Her husband's affair ended and the couple became reconciled, and Mrs J sought to remedy her enlarged girth by dieting. This only entrenched the basic cause of her overweight and set up a spiral of weight gain so rapid that, when I first saw her at the age of 36, she was over 13 stone.

Though I had known her previously, at this juncture I met her quite by chance and she invited me for a meal at her home. I noticed that she ate only very sparingly and did not join her husband and me for a drink. Later, talking to her privately, she brought up the subject of her weight and showed me a trunkful of diet books from all over the world. None had been of any help to her. She asked me if I could help her lose weight, if I knew of some magic formula or yet another crash diet which would give her back her youthful figure. She had not connected her original weight gain with her husband's infidelity, but I explained to her that this was the probable initial cause of the problem. If she had let the matter alone it would have automatically corrected itself when the affair was over, but she had compounded the problem and set up a vicious circle of weight gain by dieting. With each new diet the spiral of weight increase gained

additional momentum until now the problem was almost
intractable.

Mrs J could not understand why she remained fat when
she ate so sparingly, but soon the real reason emerged,
although it took me some time to extract it from her.
Each morning, before going to work, she would go to the
fruit market with the chauffeur and buy a massive quantity
of fruit which she would then devour in her room. In the
afternoon, after a modest lunch, she would send the
chauffeur out again for more fruit, which she would eat
before her husband came home to dinner. This was the
real cause of her overweight – she was a secret compulsive
eater. From the numerous diet books she owned, she had
gained the impression that fruit was not fattening and
satisfied her craving for food by eating large quantities
under the delusion that they would not make her fat.

Mrs J was an example of food addiction–the compulsive
eating pattern of impaired opiate release usually caused
by chronic dieting. Lack of opiate release meant that she
never achieved the satiety phenomenon and her appetite
continued to remain unsatisfied even after very large
quantities of fruit. On the Manorama Formula she began
to achieve readily identifiable sensations of satiety after
satisfying meals, and no longer felt compelled to eat fruit
between meals. She steadily lost weight and within a year
was back to her original weight of 8½ stone. She has
remained at this weight ever since.

Mrs RK, at 30, weighed 9 stone, a normal weight for her
height of 5′ 4″ and her rather large-boned build, a family
characteristic. She was an active member of a young
socialite group who were fashionably weight-conscious
and who indulged in a variety of outdoor activities in
pursuit of the fashionable figure – tennis and swimming
in the plains and mountain climbing and skating in the

mountainous regions that surrounded their town. But Mrs RK lived in a politically tense area of India, a district of Amritsar on the borders of Pakistan, where the majority of the inhabitants were Islamic, while Mrs RK's group were either Sikh or Hindu. Eventually, sectarian violence broke out and Mrs RK had to flee the district. For some time she led an unsettled life, moving from district to district, during which time she had neither the time nor the facilities for any athletic activities. She began steadily to gain weight. She dieted sporadically to combat this but always regained weight rapidly when the diet was discontinued.

When I saw Mrs RK at the age of 35, she weighed 11 stone. I introduced her to the Manorama Formula but she was difficult to persuade, being convinced that if she ate everything she wished she would gain weight rapidly. She tried the Manorama Formula three times, but each time she panicked after a few days and started dieting again. The fourth time she tried it, however, she realized that she was indeed losing weight. From then on she adhered firmly to the formula. She finally came down to under 9 stone. Mrs RK was one of my early successes. Her weight has remained stable now for nearly 15 years.

Mrs RK could be called a mild example of the 'retired athlete's syndrome' – that of weight regain after discontinuing exercise, in this case compounded by a greater food intake induced by the stress of her unsettled situation. The Manorama Formula restored her correct energy balance and her ideal weight without a return to rigorous exercise and without dieting.

Mrs Z was one of a pair of attractive twin sisters, part of a large, happy family of landowners living in one of the provinces of India. Both twins were cast in a junoesque mould, and at the age of 20 both weighed 10½ stone for a height of 5′ 6″. Mrs Z married at the age of 20. She had up to then been quite content with her statuesque proportions, and her husband gave every indication of his appreciation of her junoesque beauty. The young couple on their marriage, moved into her mother-in-law's house in New Delhi. The mother-in-law was a fashionable, sophisticated socialite. She soon resented her son's pre-occupation with his attractive young bride and began to find fault and criticize her. She herself had a very petite build, and she made constant hurtful allusions to her daughter-in-law's larger proportions. She maintained that big girls were unattractive – like 'decorated elephants' (elephants dressed up for ceremonial occasions). She declared fatness was a disease and compared an extra 10 kg of weight to carrying a 10 kg sack of flour on the head.

So Mrs Z was driven to attempting to reduce her weight. A doctor she consulted gave her pills and a diet sheet. From then on her weight followed the familiar pattern of rapid weight loss followed by still more rapid regain. It would come down to 9½ stone on rigid dieting but would then soar up to 11 stone once the diet was discarded. Her twin sister, meanwhile, remained at a constant weight of 10½ stone.

I saw Mrs Z one year later and started her on the Manorama Formula. She grasped the essentials readily, and slowly but steadily came down to 9½ stone, after which her weight remained stable. It has remained so since.

Interestingly, her twin sister also decided to follow the Manorama Formula and in due course her weight also came down to 9½ stone and remained constant thereafter.

This interesting example of twin sisters demonstrates the adverse effects of dieting in almost controlled exper-imental conditions, Mrs Z's twin being the control. Her weight remained stable without dieting whereas her sister's fluctuated wildly and eventually was only controlled by rigid food restriction. However, when Mrs Z came down to 9½ stone on the Manorama Formula her twin decided that she too wanted to come down to the same and used the Manorama Formula very effectively for this purpose. She made a conscious decision that that was the weight she wanted to be, and she was able to implement her decision easily and effortlessly by using the Manorama Formula.

Two sisters, **Mrs S** and **Mrs L,** had practically identical problems. Now in their 30s, they both had three children and both sisters, previously of normal weight, had become fat because they had failed to regain their normal weight after each pregnancy, with an average weight gain of about 10 pounds with each child. They had restricted their food intake after each birth in an effort to regain their pre-pregnancy weight more quickly. As brown fat activity is inhibited during pregnancy anyway, food restriction after the births only perpetuated this inhibition and rendered the brown fat more unreceptive to stimulation. Thus dieting in this case, as in every other, was totally counterproductive. Both sisters started following the formula at the same time, and both regained their normal weight, which they have supported to date.

These are not the dramatic stories you find in the average diet book. There was no rapid shedding of 10 pounds in one week; only a slow but steady reversion to normal weight and then stabilization at that weight.

Each of these patients' weight problems had arisen from a different cause. The sisters, Mrs S and Mrs L, demonstrate the common problem of weight gain after having children. The weight gain of pregnancy is hormonally mediated and it usually resolves itself without difficulty after the birth. But by diet restriction Mrs S and Mrs L had perpetuated the weight increase. CJ's weight gain was probably also hormonally based, occurring about the time of puberty. The problem would probably have resolved itself spontaneously, but by going on a series of drastic reducing diets it had become entrenched.

Mr K's weight gain on the other hand resulted from extraneous circumstances – the change in his lifestyle on the construction site. After a while his weight would probably have reverted to normal spontaneously, but due to the family history of hypertension he embarked on a diet which, by inhibiting brown fat activity and slowing up his metabolism, paved the way for his eventual chronic obesity problem.

Mrs L's weight gain of 20 pounds was not a large one but she was devoted to the fashionable ideal of the very slender figure, and so began the progression to chronic weight problems. This has been the cause of many women's destabilization of their weight-control mechanism. Many women go on a diet when they are already of normal weight in order to be able to wear some particular dress or for some particular occasion, thus setting the scene for the progression from diet to diet without success, and with increasing weight gain and destabilization of the control mechanism.

I could recount many other case histories. But most of the people I saw had given up the struggle with their weight and had resigned themselves to permanent fatness. If pressurized by the family, they made half-hearted attempts at dieting, even though they never ate very large meals in any case. Many had run the gamut of every new crash diet that made its appearance – the single-item diets, the fruit diets, the boiled meat only diets, the all-protein diets. They were now discouraged, depressed, and obsessed with their weight problem, but at the same time helpless to know how to relieve it. Many had reached the stage where their whole lives were blighted by the constant battle.

It was these depressed and discouraged patients who proved so rewarding to treat. Their reduction to normal weight was achieved painlessly and easily. They were able to enjoy their food for the first time for many years, without guilt and anxiety. It was a truly liberating experience. Many were now able to eat with the family for the first time without feeling envious or deprived. They were able to socialize freely and eat and drink at parties as much as they wished. The whole experience had the most remarkable effect on their character, personality and outlook on life. From the lethargic, depressed people I first met there emerged vigorous, happy people bounding in life and energy. For these people the Manorama Formula changed their lives. It can do the same for you.

11
Universal application

This book made you a promise – that you would attain perfect weight control; that you would have it permanently; that you would be freed from perpetual concern about your weight.

Now this book makes you a further, fundamental promise: that you can gain perfect control over all your other vital instincts and freedom from concern with them. By following the principles of the Manorama Formula, you can gain the same degree of control over these instincts as you did with the instinct to eat.

The instinct to eat to nourish, the instinct to sleep to recuperate, the instinct to have sex and propagate, are all essential for the sustenance of life. The instinct to move, to seek food, to find shelter and obtain objects to make the shelter habitable, where food and rest can be enjoyed and secured, to find a sexual partner with whom to share the enjoyment of food, comfort, rest and the rewards of labour, is also basic. The instinct to move supports the instincts which sustain life, i.e. the instincts to eat, sleep and have sex for the purpose of the propagation of the species.

These basic instincts essential to survival we possess in common with the animal kingdom. However, man has a rational brain, and possesses the ability to gain mastery over his instincts. The way to gain control of your instincts is through their perfect fulfilment; when you have achieved perfect fulfilment they will serve you rather than enslave you.

Starting from the common ground of the instincts basic

to survival, when you have learnt to fulfil them perfectly, you will be free to progress further. You will spontaneously develop the will to excel and you will excel. You will then automatically progress to the next stage and develop your individual personality in terms of the higher activities, i.e. inventiveness, creativity, adventure and spirituality. You will be free to express your uniqueness.

In the last analysis, this book is about freedom, freedom to develop and assert your uniqueness, which is your birthright and purpose of life.

As the progress of individual development is dependent on physical well-being, which in turn is dependent on the proper fulfilment of the vital instincts, nature has not left this to chance. It has made provision for their perfect fulfilment. It has endowed them with an infallible, chemically mediated reward system – the release of the natural opiates that occurs when they are fulfilled.

Opiate release is the common denominator of the physiological pleasure gained from all these instincts. The nature of the pleasure may be different in each instinct; but the physiological basis in the release of the opiates is the same, whether it is reflected in the feeling of uplift and exhilaration gained from physical activity, the lowering of tension induced by sleep and rest during the day, or the pleasure of sex which is at once both exhilarating and tension-releasing.

The regular and sufficient release of these opiates, which is indicated by the accompanying arousal of physiological pleasure, is the only criterion by which the efficient execution of these instincts can be realized. Whatever the instinct, it can only be properly fulfilled in response to the inner signals from the body. Inner signals will never go away. When they are interfered with by outside dictates, there will be conflict; the release of opiates will be diminished. When the signals are ignored, the release of opiates will be erratic. Either way, the result will be frustration of the instinct. Whichever instinct they are concerned with, external dictates are counterproductive, damaging and dangerous; by precluding the normal release of the opiates they can induce vulnerability to various chemical addictions.

Nature has provided the equipment for pleasure – complete systems for the proper fulfilment of the instincts, distinct anatomical systems with their own neurochemical transmission circuits. These individual systems all carry the potential to generate chemically mediated pleasure through their abundant supply of opiates. The opiates give us freedom from external sources of pleasure. All that is necessary to allow them their full potential is to respond to them and safeguard them from outside interference.

If the basic instincts are properly fulfilled, there will, in the ordinary course of the day, be a 24-hour supply of opiates available, through eating, walking, sleeping and relaxing. There is a perfect dispersal system which dissipates the opiates when they have fulfilled their purpose, creating a demand for further release through the execution of the instincts. The system provides a perfectly balanced variation of heightening and dampening down of excitation. This guarantees pleasure throughout the day and protects you from vulnerability to lack of pleasure.

Each instinct arises in cycles, according to the internal clock, in such a way that there is normally no overlap. By focussing on the signals of that instinct exclusively, the finer tuning of the clock is preserved. The clock makes provision for a recurring supply of opiates throughout the day.

You are now familiar with the power of physiological pleasure. You will have learnt that physiological pleasure is not just the familiar subjective feelings of pleasure, comfort and ease, but that these are reflections of a force generated by special physiological systems with distinct anatomical foundations. These anatomical systems are exclusively connected with a specific instinct. In the instinct to nourish, you took account of your inner signals and responded to their messages, thereby ensuring efficient execution of that instinct. You knew you were executing it efficiently because you generated the power of physiological pleasure. You knew you had generated this power because you felt its subjective accompaniments – the cluster of pleasurable feelings that arose. The test of the efficient execution of any instinct of survival is whether or not it leads to these sensations.

Only you and you alone are able to make this assessment. Only your own inner signals can guide you in making it. No externally directed dictates can accomplish it.

When you have understood the significance of pleasure and pain, you will be able to exploit the full potential of pleasure, which is inherently linked, not only with the instinct to nourish, but equally with all other vital instincts.

The importance of painful sensations can never be minimized. Nature does not tolerate pain. If there are both pleasurable and painful sensations present at the same time, pain will have precedence.

The role of pleasure is to promote life. The role of pain is to preserve life. Life can be promoted by pleasure only after it has been preserved by the elimination of pain. Painful sensations are emergency warnings that carry the message that life or well-being is under threat; they carry too the corollary demand that the causative factor must be removed, neutralized or dispersed.

When a bone is broken, pain conveys the necessity of

immobilization to eliminate further damage. It will prevent movement towards a goal no matter how desirable that goal may be. When there is internal obstruction or inflammation in any vital system, pain conveys the necessity for immediate action to rectify the situation.

All actions carry an overall capacity to evoke pleasurable or painful responses. If your desire or aim is to be fulfilled, it must be a procedure which is pleasurable. To be consistent, pleasure can only become operative in the absence of pain.

Pleasure is not only a constant source of power – it has a constant nature as well.

It is in the nature of pleasure that it has a momentum of its own.

Any procedure which is pleasurable will proceed on its own momentum.

Any procedure which is pleasurable is self-promoting.

Any procedure which is pleasurable will propel you towards your goal.

Once initiated, any procedure which is pleasurable will continue to propel you towards your goal until that goal is achieved.

It is in the nature of pleasure that it is self-perpetuating.

You can chemically induce pleasure whenever you wish by the perfect fulfilment of the instincts.

The instinct for upright posture and movement, without which you could not survive, is inherent. Movement fulfils the basic survival needs of the body in the search for food, a place to recuperate, and a life partner. If efficiently executed, it carries enormous potential for physiological pleasure and its subjective accompaniments of ease, comfort and mood uplift. Sports and other physical activities are also accompanied by opiate release and so generate physiological pleasure. It is this potential that is exploited by the leisure industry.

The potential for pleasure from the instinct to move lies in the body itself. The more this potential is developed, the less your dependence on the commercial pressures of the leisure industry and its promotion of a concept of 'fitness' linked with some particular product or regime. The blanket concept of 'fitness' has no relevance to your internal signals. Without regard to your inner signals, the promotion of pleasure by any particular regime will be problematic. You can obtain a full measure of pleasure from physical activity with certainty, and during the ordinary course of your day, by following your own inner signals. Efficient use of your muscular system during the course of your day-to-day activities will generate vitality without resorting to imposed exercise regimes. By regularly following the guidance from the signals arising from your own skeletomuscular system, your discerning powers will become so finely tuned that you will be able to make the optimal choice of the additional physical activity which will be the most fulfilling for you, which will best accord with your own particular preference and bodily needs, and you will naturally come to know whether you would derive most pleasure from carrying it out alone, in company, or in competition and in what surroundings.

Blanket claims for the benefits of exercise are unscientific. Whether the activity is beneficial or not will depend on its sensory component. If you are generating physiological pleasure, you are using your muscular system efficiently, and this will be reflected in the comfort and mood uplift you experience. That is the real benefit. There is no other benefit arising from fitness. If you are not generating this pleasure, you will not only cause exhaustion and wear and tear, but you will be subjecting yourself to other risks. The crucial element is the PP factor, which you can only generate by disregarding external dictates.

You can use your instinct to move and have perfect

posture and muscle tone while you walk, stand, sit or even while you sleep, with the same efficiency and harmony as you did with your instinct to nourish. You can do this and achieve precise muscle control in the ordinary course of your daily activities. It will spill over its benefits to the entire body. The Hunza community, the second longest-living community in the world, subsists on sub-standard food and yet walk miles each day in search of this food. They not only live to be over 100, their women regularly produce normal children in their sixties. The Hunzas owe their health and vigour largely to the fact that they have perfected their individual posture and rhythm in walking.

The bulk of the body is made up of voluntary muscles which subserve posture and movement. The muscles, each of which has a sensory component, transmit impulses to the brain, which exercises overall control.

Unlike the instincts to nourish, to sleep and to have sex, which arise in cycles, the impulses from the muscles serving posture and movement are transmitted continuously throughout the day and to some extent at night also. Consequently, this instinct carries the most sustained potential for physiological pleasure or for pain in comparison with any other vital instinct.

Posture is maintained by two opposing muscle groups acting reciprocally. A group of muscles becomes tense when a maximum number of nervous impulses are being transmitted; it is relaxed only when a minimum number are involved. In the postures of sitting or standing, the two opposing groups of muscles are brought into play. If there were an imbalance of tension in these muscles, then the body would tilt in the direction where there was more supportive tension. Therefore, posture is physiologically correct when there is an equal number of impulses in both groups. Whether your body is relaxed or tense will depend on the number of impulses. Your body will be physiologically upright and relaxed when both opposing groups are transmitting equally, with a minimal number of impulses.

Perfect posture is personal and individual. As no two people have an identical body build, neither do they have an identical perfect posture. You can attain your perfect posture no matter what the circumstances by identifying the inner signals arising from your muscles. You can respond to tension from any group of muscles by voluntary change to a position where these signals cease to arise. This cannot be done by outside dictates. It can only be done by identifying and neutralizing the signals. So perfect posture can be achieved by identifying the inner signals of tension and altering the muscular position in response. When all tension has been neutralized, physiological pleasure will have been generated. You will recognize this by the corresponding subjective feelings of comfort, ease and pleasure.

This is exactly the same principle as you applied to the instinct to nourish, that is, you paid regard to your inner signals and took the voluntary action which led to the generation of physiological pleasure.

Perfect rhythm of movement is individual. No two people have an identical rhythm. Movement too is conducted by two opposing groups of muscles acting reciprocally. If an external movement is performed in obedience to the inner signals and the muscles are moved in a manner which gives rise to a minimal amount of tension, this minimal tension is indicative of the efficiency of the movement and will generate physiological pleasure.

The test again is the subjective feelings of pleasure and comfort generated. Most people instinctively acquire a reasonable posture and rhythm of movement. When, however, a posture is taken up in response to external dictates, as in exercise workouts, they are bound to conflict with the inner signals. And if negative signals are ignored, wear and tear of the tissues, and possibly, damage, will result. Aerobic exercises can cause wear and tear, aging of the muscles, and the risk of permanent damage to the skeletomuscular system. Jogging carries the same potential for harm if bodily signals of pain and exhaustion are ignored.

Physiological pleasure is not only a specific power, it is also specifically different when different sets of muscles are brought into play. It is different when they are brought into play at different speeds whatever the activity.

Walkers who have learnt to generate physiological pleasure experience an accompanying subjective mood uplift of a specific nature. They often describe their subjective feelings in terms of being at peace with themselves. You can achieve the same feeling on your way to work or in working in your house. When the rules of generating physiological pleasure are obeyed, jogging is accompanied by a different kind of mood uplift, described by many as 'euphoric'. Golf, because of the precision of stance and movement which the game requires, generates physiological pleasure out of proportion to the amount of actual exercise involved. Many golfers, in fact, describe being 'addicted' to the game. When all these activities are performed efficiently, there is release of the natural opiates. The positive subjective feelings that ensue from the release of opiates indicate that they are being performed with perfect posture and rhythm of movement and hence generating physiological pleasure.

The instinct to recuperate entails the slowing down of all bodily activities in the setting of sleep, and the periodic slowing down of these activities within the course of the day.

In nature, opiates are released according to the internal clock, inducing sleep at night and periodic relaxation during the day. All this is perfectly matched to your body's need to recuperate. The opiates effect lowering of mental and physical activity and generate pleasure in response to these needs. All that it is necessary for you to do to achieve the maximum benefit from the instinct to recuperate is to heed the inner signals that arise in response to your internal clock.

Sleeping tablets produce the dampening down of bodily and mental activity by chemical means, an artificial process which mimics the action of the natural opiates. But with sleeping drugs, the normal dispersal system of the opiates is absent and the drug effects persist into the next day. The introduction of artificial chemicals into the system precludes the generation of opiates and sets up a vicious circle of insomnia.

Most people recuperate reasonably well through sleep. There is, however, a great deal of variation in the quality of sleep, which is reflected in health and vitality.

Normal sleep is a process whereby external interactions are cut off and internal activities minimized. Therefore, all stimuli of sound, sight, and pressure on the body should be minimized. You will then minimize the impulses from the muscles as you did in the case of sitting and standing. In lying down, a minimal number of impulses are necessary to support your posture. So in lying down also, you should take note of tension in any group of muscles and voluntarily change your position in response, until you start generating physiological pleasure. In fact, you apply the same principles in lying down in your bed as you applied to sitting and standing. The object is to reduce the impulses arising from the muscles to an absolute minimum and produce maximum opiate release.

Most people in the West do not attain a reasonable degree of physical relaxation during the course of the day. They fail to respond to the inner signals of tension which demand relaxation. These signals arise periodically, and by the release of opiates can be relieved in a matter of minutes. If they are ignored, however, tension escalates and requires a disproportionately longer period to relieve, making you vulnerable to tranquillizers and excess of alcohol. Consistent disregard leads to chronic fatigue and other symptoms of ill health. Relaxation in an awake setting can be attained in a matter of minutes provided it is in response to the internal clock which provides for prompt opiate release in response to the body's inner demands.

By this time you will have already learnt to relax and generate physiological pleasure from your muscular system. You will be able simultaneously to reduce the activity of your inner systems. All you need do now is to learn to reduce your mental activity. The ancient Indian practice of *barhas*, known in the West as transcendental meditation, is a simple technique producing a special kind of relaxation beneficial to every system in the body. It is achieved by focussing your attention on a particular object, image or sound. It is normal for this focus to shift away from the object. All you have to do is repeatedly to bring it back into focus. When you have done this a few times you will, in a matter of minutes, experience tangible feelings of increased vitality. Contrary to the claims of many purveyors of transcendental meditation in the West, who demand that a personal mantra be prescribed for each individual, the principle of the technique is the repetition of the focussing; the choice of the object of focus is in itself irrelevant. In India, where transcendental meditation has been practised for centuries, no such stipulation is ever made. The only stipulation is that it is never taught for money.

Like the instinct to stand upright and walk, the instinct for sex, once having matured, can continue throughout life. Members of some South American and Australian aboriginals regularly have sex more than once a night. In contrast, semi-celibate communities have sex on rare occasions for the purpose of having children only. They are able to do this by excluding environmental stimuli in such a way that opiates are not released.

With the appropriate stimulus, opiates are released and arousal heightened. When sufficient opiates are released and sufficient pleasure has been gained, there is an automatic switch-off mechanism which comes into force. Further release of opiates and arousal is inhibited. Rebound relaxation takes place. All systems are relaxed. Instinct arousal is inhibited until the next cycle.

The instinct for sex arises regularly and automatically. As long as the response is pleasurable it produces opiates leading to instinct fulfilment. Conversely, unpleasurable responses to the inner signals weaken the signals by biofeedback mechanisms. Weaker inner signals can be revitalized at any time by appropriate pleasurable responses.

As in the instinct to eat, imagination is the natural link between arousal of inner signals and fulfilment of the sex instinct. It takes into account the realistic options available, past pleasant experiences, the moral confines, and selects the right means of instinct fulfilment. It also instinctively selects the most appropriate modes of fulfilment. Imagery leads to practice.

Imagery is not only a crucial link between instinct arousal in the body and instinct fulfilment, it is the foundation stone of individual future direction. It is the forerunner of planned self-determination. It unleashes the secondary instincts special to man, namely, adventure, and enterprise. It promotes the highest mental, creative and spiritual capabilities.

You have the detailed model of the efficient fulfilment

of the instinct to eat before you. You know all instincts arise naturally. You know that if you respond to the inner signals in a way that induces pleasure, it will then be opiate-mediated. The release of opiates will automatically reinforce pleasure and culminate in satiety at all levels. You know that in due course, pleasure will become programmed in the cortex. It will then automatically reproduce the right response at the right time. The cortex will then be freed from involvement with the basic mechanics of the instincts of survival.

Freed by automatic, continuous pleasure from instinct fulfilment, your brain will achieve its true potential. Your mind and body will work in perfect harmony with the maximum productivity. All your goals will be achieved. You will be totally free.

Appendix

The Manorama Formula
reproduced under controlled conditions

Pleasure is not just a transient subjective sensation. It has a physical substructure with a complicated system of nervous circuits and chemical substances in the body to support it. Because pleasure is important to the survival of the species; without pleasure, eating to sustain life would become a duty to be performed conscientiously by the dutiful but sporadically by the careless, like cleaning the teeth, for example. For animals, there would be no concept even of its necessity, no feelings of duty such as exist in man. But a regular daily intake of food in measured quantities to provide a continuous supply of energy and to repair tissues is necessary to sustain life.

So nature had to build in a powerful reward system specifically centred around the ingestion of food. It contrived this by building in a whole range of pleasures centred around eating, pleasures of sight, smell, texture and taste. It had to ensure that this pleasure was of sufficient intensity to maintain life and health. It also had to ensure that *not* eating caused active *dis*pleasure. Thus it also built in sensations of hunger and thirst of sufficient urgency to demand speedy satisfaction.

It was also important that pleasure in eating should be counterbalanced by *dis*pleasure in *over*eating, that there should be a built-in switch-off mechanism which tells the animal that it has eaten enough to fulfil its bodily needs. If there were no switch-off mechanism the animal, having no means to measure its food intake, would continue to eat until the whole system became overloaded. So along with a reward system for the ingestion of food, a system signalling satiety had to be built in. This we know as the familiar feeling of satiety when we have had a good meal, the feeling when food formerly pleasurable becomes actively displeasurable when enough has been ingested.

The precision with which the system operates is awesome. One has only to watch a herd of cattle, a flock of sheep, a flight of birds, or even a hive of bees to realize its almost mathematical accuracy. All these birds and animals are of almost uniform size. Without this precise system of weight control this uniformity would be impossible. Man too possesses innate, in-built weight control. Its precision is emphasized by the recent estimation that the average woman gains only 11 kg between the ages of 25 and 65, during which time she has eaten 20 tons of food – a weight change corresponding to an average daily error of only 350 mg of food.

The extreme accuracy of the control of intake to match precisely the body's size has been demonstrated in laboratory experiments with rats in which the standard laboratory diet was replaced by one diluted with a non-food filler, like bran, so that the actual calorie content was reduced from 2.8 to 1.5 per gram while the bulk remained the same. The rats promptly increased their intake in exact proportion to the dilution of the diet. A converse experiment was performed in which the calorie content of the diet was raised to 5.1 calories per gram by adding suet. The rats reduced their intake in exact proportion to the added suet.

It is now generally accepted that the overall control of bodily weight is located in an organ in the brain called the hypothalamus. This location is supported by laboratory experiments in which lesions made in part of this organ in experimental animals have rendered them obese. Relays of information from different parts of the body are passed to the hypothalamus by regulatory feed-back mechanisms. In response the hypothalamus sends out signals to the areas concerned with feeding. This implies that accurate assessments of energy needs are being made somewhere in the body before being passed to the hypothalamus. Some mechanism must therefore exist for assessing the size of the fat stores in the body by a comprehensive system of sensing. The identity of the sensing mechanism is not yet known, but it is believed to be hormonal, or hormone-mediated. Administration of steroid hormones leads to a rise in body weight and fat content. This is the reason for the weight gain on the 'pill' so often reported. Weight gain during pregnancy is also hormonally mediated.

Supportive evidence for the hormone theory arises from experiments with 'parabiotic rats'. These are surgically united pairs of rats which therefore share a common blood supply. If one rat is made obese by lesions in the hypothalamus, the other reduces its food intake and becomes very thin, evidently in response to the obesity of its partner.

Modern scientific experiments have demonstrated that weight control, as far as food ingestion and satiety are concerned, begins and ends with the sense of taste. In order that the switch-off mechanism could operate efficiently, nature had to build in a mechanism whereby the taste which was so pleasurable at the start of a meal became actively displeasurable when enough food was ingested. This was proved experimentally by the American scientist M. Cabanac and his team in a series of experiments in the 1970s. The team used themselves as experimental subjects. After a period of total fasting, they were given samples of a sweet solution to taste and asked to rate it for pleasantness or unpleasantness on a scale of 1 to 5. All rated the samples pleasant. However, after ingesting a large quantity of glucose and then being given the same samples, all rated them as unpleasant. A similar experiment was performed for the sense of smell. Sniffing an orange syrup was found to be pleasant by fasting subjects, but after an ingestion of a large glucose load it became unpleasant. So taste can actually change in relation to the body's needs. A particular taste which seems pleasurable in one situation can actually become unpleasurable in another. The experiments were interpreted by Cabanac as evidence that the taste and smell of food is directly controlled by the inner signals of the body. 'Pleasure,' he said, 'is a signal of usefulness and displeasure is a signal of the absence of any need.' So pleasure is an important indication of the body's needs.

An earlier experiment by Cabanac had produced similar alterations in the sensation of temperature in response to the inner signals of the body. A subject placed in a bath of water was asked to rate the pleasurableness or otherwise of different temperatures. The responses varied according to the subject's own internal temperature. When the bath water was warm a cool stimulus was rated as pleasant. When the water was made cold, the same stimulus was rated as unpleasant. 'Pleasure occurs,' Cabanac concluded, 'whenever a sensation indicates the presence of a stimulus which helps to correct an internal trouble.' So here again the *inner signals* of the body prevailed.

Cabanac's conclusion from his tasting experiment was that taste could be monitored by *internal signals* from the body which indicate its precise needs from hour to hour, signals which override the sense of taste itself. Nature contrived this adaptability of the senses as a means of controlling intake. He suspected that the adaptability of the sense of taste was related to some regulatory factor governing not only food ingestion but also weight control.

To establish this, Cabanac performed further experiments. His team, all of normal weight, underwent a reduced calorie diet, reducing their food intake to 500 or 800 calories per day until they had reduced their body weight by 10 per cent. During this period of weight reduction, the ability of the sense of taste to change from pleasant to unpleasant after a load of glucose disappeared completely. Ingestion of as much as 50 grams of glucose was insufficient to render the stimuli unpleasant. When the subjects returned to their normal body weight, however, the ability of the taste sensations to change from pleasant to unpleasant was fully restored. He repeated his experiments with obese subjects and found that in every case these subjects had lost their ability to alter taste sensations from pleasant to unpleasant after ingestion of a glucose load. 'This would suggest that obesity is a resetting of the ponderostat [a name he coined for the setting of the weight control mechanism] at a higher body weight,' he wrote. 'If the obese person, for health or social reasons, combats his obesity, he will lower his body weight below the set "obese" level.' The ability to change his taste sensations would disappear and satiety would be impaired. He concluded from his experiments that the central weight-control mechanism in the body must be as constant as the body's regulation of temperature.

The changing of a given taste stimulus from pleasure to displeasure is the key factor in the body's regulation of food intake to match its energy needs and those of overall weight control. It is the signal of satiety that tells us forcibly and unequivocally that we have eaten enough. As we have seen, this response is controlled by overriding inner signals from the body. In the obese individual, these inner signals have been blunted; he has either lost touch with them or has not paid sufficient attention to them. So he has got fat.

Since Cabanac performed his classic experiments, much new information has emerged, and the remaining pieces in the complex puzzle of weight control have come to light. While underlining Cabanac's original assumptions, they have demonstrated the important fact that before satiety is achieved, you must first gain pleasure from eating. Before your taste can change from pleasure to displeasure you must first have pleasure.

Pleasure is the trigger that implements the decisions of the weight-control mechanism – pleasure in the sight, smell and taste of food. It is not pleasure in eating that causes obesity – it is insufficient pleasure in eating.

So if we are to arouse the signals of satiety in order to operate the switch-off mechanism, we must first derive the maximum amount of pleasure from our food. We must ensure that it is highly palatable, that it is the food we want to eat at that particular time of day, and that it conforms to the demands of the inner signals emanating from our bodies. We ignore our inner signals when we eat lettuce and cottage cheese on a cold day when we hunger for a hot, appetizing dish. We ignore our inner signals when we deprive ourselves of salt and other condiments and eat flavourless, tasteless dishes to comply with the latest food theory. We ignore our inner signals when we go on any calorie-restriction diet. If we ignore our inner signals for too long, in time they become blunted and fail to serve us as pointers to health and weight control.

Taste and palatability have another important function for weight control. Eating the food of choice from a range of highly palatable foods is one of the two stimuli that activates the brown fat we referred to in Chapter 3 Rats allowed to eat freely from a variety of palatable foods (the 'cafeteria diet') were found to have enhanced brown fat activity, in contrast to control rats given the ordinary laboratory 'chow'. The food offered, besides being palatable, was frequently varied to maintain interest.

Nature's reward system for the ingestion of food had to be precise in its functioning. It had not only to reward food intake but it had to reward intake of the right kind. Food does not come in the wild pre-packed with all the essential ingredients for good nutritional balance. There had to be an in-built system enabling the animal to select precisely from the nutrients available to it the exact food elements needed to provide the essential nutrients to sustain life and health.

Man also possesses this in-built mechanism. The modern science of nutrition is little more than 100 years old. Many important food elements essential for the maintenance of life, the vitamins, the essential amino acids, some of the trace elements, for example, have only been discovered in the past 50 years. Yet man has survived for thousands of years without any knowledge of proteins, carbohydrates, vitamins and minerals. Before any scientific nutritional information was formulated, man was making the correct nutritional decisions. How did he do this? He did it entirely through his own in-built mechanisms for assessing the nutritional quality of the food available to him. This information came to him through his senses and through the pleasure he derived from eating particular foods at particular times of day and in particular situations. The fact that man has survived for thousands of years using only these sources of information presupposes an awesome precision in the guidance afforded him through the pleasures of his senses.

At its most elementary, taste guided both man and animals to avoid poisonous berries and plants and to eat only those harmless to the body. But taste had to be far more precise than this. It had to indicate the need for the specific nutrients the body requires from time to time for its optimal well-being. We have seen that it does this more precisely than any of the nutritional guidelines produced today. Conflicting dietary advice, food superstitions, food taboos, have all conspired to blunt the finer tuning of man's response to his inner signals, and to learn about this tuning at its most awesome we have to resort to veterinary literature and to laboratory animal experiments.

There are a number of reports in agricultural journals which show that animals allowed to choose their food freely show selection abilities that lead to normal or above normal health, growth and reproduction. In these studies it was noted that as young animals mature they select a diet of increasing protein and energy content. Chickens reared on a dietary self-selection regime grew better and produced a higher egg yield. In one experiment, cows allowed to graze freely from four haystacks ate exclusively from the one stack composed of hay grown on fertilized soil. Chemical analysis showed that the chosen hay was of better nutritional quality than the other hay. W. Godden, while analysing the mineral composition of various pasture lands in Britain, noted the mineral make-up of the grasses to be the most nutritionally adequate. In the phosphorus-poor grazing land of South Africa, cattle became bone eaters to satisfy their phosphorus requirements. The addition of phosphorus to their diet put an end to the practice. An appetite for bone has also been reported in pregnant and lactating grey squirrels.

The innate nutritional wisdom of animals in food selection was studied intensively by C.P. Richter, who performed a classic series of experiments on laboratory rats in whom he removed different organs governing different metabolic functions of the body, thereby studying the rats' compensatory food choices.

Removal of the adrenal glands disturbs sodium metabolism and sodium is lost from the body in large quantities. When this was performed on rats fed the stock laboratory diet they died in 8 to 18 days. When permitted free access by Richter to a salt solution, they took a sufficient quantity to remain alive and symptom-free. Similarly, rats whose parathyroid gland (the gland that controls calcium metabolism) was removed they developed tetany, a symptom of calcium deficiency, on the stock diet. When given free access to a calcium solution, however, they took enough to remain alive and free from tetany. When parathyroid tissue was implanted, the rats at once reduced their calcium intake to normal. Removal of the posterior lobe of the pituitary gland disturbs the regulation of water metabolism. Large amounts of urine are excreted and animals so inflicted soon die if water is restricted. Richter's rats, however, given free access to water, ingested large amounts and remained in good health.

Richter's studies of pregnancy and lactation in rats demonstrated the remarkable precision of the rats' innate capacity to regulate food intake to meet changing metabolic requirements. His results showed an increase in sodium chloride intake during the first five days of pregnancy, a further increase in the second half of the lactation period, and a prompt return to normal intake with weaning. Calcium intake increased slightly during pregnancy and markedly during lactation (30–40 times the intake before mating). After weaning, intake returned to the original level only after several weeks. A similar pattern was established with the appetite for sodium phosphate. Appetite for protein and fat increased slightly during pregnancy and more during lactation, but decreased rapidly after weaning. Carbohydrate intake remained essentially unchanged. The most interesting observation, however, was that while rats on the stock laboratory diet and those on the self-selected diet produced the same number of young, and maintained them in good health during the nursing period, the rats selecting their own diet took 20 per cent less food in grams during pregnancy and almost 50 per cent less at the height of lactation. Richter explained this by the fact that these animals could obtain the essential elements of nutrition without taking other less-needed foodstuffs in large amounts.

A recently performed experiment demonstrated the precision with which rats adapted their food choice to a metabolic condition. A number of rats were artificially rendered diabetic with injections of streptozotocin (a substance which destroys the pancreas thus artificially inducing diabetes). They displayed all the classic symptoms of diabetes, including polydipsia (increased thirst) and polyuria (increased output of urine) and had sugar in their urine (glycosuria) as well as raised blood sugar levels (hyperglycaemia). Allowed a free choice of food, the rats automatically adapted their diets to consume more protein and less carbohydrate than non-diabetic rats. This pattern of diet brought about a reduction of the diabetic symptoms. There was decreased polyuria, polydipsia and glycosuria. Their blood sugar levels came down. In contrast, other diabetic rats consuming the composite 'rat chow' laboratory diet, experienced a steady increase in their diabetic symptoms. Further, the degree to which diabetic rats increased their protein and fat consumption was exactly matched to the severity of the disease. Later, the rats consuming the composite 'chow', which is low in fat and high in carbohydrate, began to overeat to increase their intake of fat, a readily utilizable fuel in diabetes. The free choice animals did not overeat. Yet it has taken more than a century for human beings to work out the optimal diet in diabetes. These animals, knowing nothing of proteins, carbohydrates or fats, automatically selected the right diet in the right quantities.

The precision of the 'specific hungers' possessed by animals is strikingly demonstrated by the experiments in the free selection of protein substances. These showed that rats prefer complete or balanced amino acid diets to those in which the amino acid content was imbalanced or when it lacked an essential amino acid (the component of metabolized protein which repairs worn-out muscle tissue). This innate wisdom was also demonstrated for vitamin intake. When rats were given a vitamin B-deficient diet they increased their intake of fat and decreased their consumption of carbohydrate. A fatty diet is vitamin B-sparing, as this vitamin is an essential co-enzyme for carbohydrate metabolism.

That the role of *taste* was the mediator in all these dietary choices was demonstrated by Richter. In an effort to establish the basis of the self-regulatory activity, he found that sectioning of all the taste nerves abolished the animal's ability to make beneficial dietary selections, indicating taste as the primary factor governing these choices. He concluded that taste thresholds vary with internal needs, and in a further experiment discovered that rats distinguish sodium chloride solutions from water in concentrations as low as 1:2000, but that adrenalecto-mized rats can distinguish it in solutions of *as low as 1:33,000*. He was convinced that beneficial selections depend on taste alone, and neither on experience or on the physiological effects produced by the substance.

Thus, Professor Richter showed that a pronounced physiological need may lower the taste threshold for the required substance so markedly that it can be detected in minute quantities. This was dramatically demonstrated in the case of rats kept on a diet deficient in vitamin B; these rats were able to distinguish the bottle containing the vitamin B replacement from as many as 12 containers of other solutions and food. They ate the vitamin B greedily and clung to the bottle with paws and teeth if an attempt was made to remove it.

These experiments were made on rats. But rats have traditionally been used in nutrition studies because of the fact that the nutrient requirements of rats and human beings are essentially the same, apart from vitamin C (rats, in common with most other animals and unlike man, have the ability to synthesize their own vitamin C and are thus independent of external sources of the vitamin). Professor Richter additionally established that rats have almost identical taste thresholds to humans. The average concentration of salt in solution before it becomes recognizable he found was 0.065 in humans and 0.055 in rats, for instance. In the case of the bitter-tasting toxic compound phenylthiocarbamide, however, there was an even closer correspondence – the threshold was exactly the same for rats as it was for humans.

But Professor Richter went on to perform human experiments which conclusively demonstrated that man has the same inherent ability as animals to make beneficiary dietary selections. As he appositely pointed out, the fact that we have the same ability is attested by our very existence. In the wild state, he said, 'man did not have the guiding hand of the modern nutritionist to help him select his diet. Appetite must have been his chief guide then, and today appetite must still play a far more important role than many nutritionists seem willing to admit.'

In an experiment with 328 school children, Richter found that at 5 years of age 100 per cent of girls and 92 per cent of boys liked the taste of cod liver oil when it was offered to them. With advancing age, progressively fewer liked it, until at 14 years only 36 per cent of boys and 28 per cent of girls liked it. The appetite of these children for cod liver oil corresponded perfectly to their physiological need for the vitamin D contained in it. In the rapid phase of growth before puberty, when the size of the bony skeleton is increasing at a greater rate, the need for vitamin D, which is essential to the metabolism of calcium, is high. After puberty, when the rate is slower, the need for the vitamin is progressively reduced.

That the modern human infant is capable of selecting a diet which provides well for his nutritional needs was demonstrated by the American physician, Dr C. Davis. To a group of newly weaned children aged 8 to 10 months, she presented 35 kinds of simple complete foods from which they were allowed to select freely without any attempt being made to guide their choice. The experiment was continued for six and twelve-month periods, and in each case it was found that the child's selection had resulted in excellent nutrition as evidenced by growth, weight, bone development, musculature, general vigour, and appearance of health and well-being.

It is of special interest in this experiment that cod liver oil and a milk containing it were included routinely in the foods offered to one of the children, who had had active rickets at the beginning of the experiment. During the early months of the trial, this child voluntarily consumed from these foods a total of 258 cc of cod liver oil in 101 days. He stopped his consumption of them at the identical time that his blood calcium and phosphorus levels had become restored to normal levels and the monthly X-ray showed that the rickets had been healed.

Professor Richter also found evidence from the 'experiments of nature' that man shares with animals the ability to make beneficial selections of food guided by taste alone. In various diseases where the physiological regulators have been either completely or partially eliminated, he found the same beneficiary compensatory alterations in taste. Thus, in Addison's disease, in which there is destruction of the cortex, or the outside covering of the adrenal glands, with a consequent high rate of salt loss from the body, Professor Richter found that many of these patients had a marked craving for salt or for foods with a high salt content such as ham, sauerkraut, etc. One patient, a 34-year-old man with advanced Addison's disease, put a ⅛-inch layer of salt on his steak and used nearly half a glass of salt for his tomato juice. He used salt on oranges and grapefruit and even made lemonade with salt. Richter described the case of one patient, a 3½-year-old boy suffering from disease of the adrenal glands, who kept himself alive for more than two years by eating large amounts of salt, literally by the handful. When his salt intake was restricted to the amounts present in a normal hospital diet, he promptly developed symptoms of insufficiency and died. So remarkable was the salt-appetite in these patients that Richter considered the appearance of this symptom should raise the diagnostic possibility of disease of the adrenal glands.

Similarly, children with parathyroid deficiency, which interferes with calcium metabolism, have been reported to show a craving for chalk, plaster and other substances with a high calcium content. Instances have been reported in which patients with pernicious anaemia have developed a strong craving for liver and have kept themselves in good health by satisfying the desire. Professor Richter believed that dietary anaemias may be the cause of the common practice of clay-eating prevalent in the poor sections of South American states. The iron contained in the clay remedied the deficiencies of their dietary intake, he found. The high water intake of patients with diabetes insipidus Richter believed to be an effort to prevent dehydration, which is threatened by the loss of the

physiological regulatory water balance action of the posterior lobe of the pituitary gland. Similarly, the voracious
appetite of hyperthyroid patients he attributed directly to
the increased metabolic rate produced by overactivity of
the gland, which would result in semi-starvation if the
food intake were limited to normal amounts.

Professor Richter, presenting all this data in his dis-
tinguished Harvey Lecture, affirmed his conviction that
they demonstrated that the ability to select diets that
satisfied internal needs depends more upon taste sensation
than on experience, and that humans possess this faculty
in common with animals. 'We believe the results of our
experiments indicate that in human beings and animals
the effort to maintain a constant internal environment
constitutes one of the most universal and powerful of all
behaviour urges or drives,' he said.

Following the dictates of your own appetite-hunger-
taste signals makes sound nutritional sense. The Manorama Formula is not only a blueprint for weight control
but one for optimal nutrition as well.

The formula is thus of benefit not only to those who
want to lose weight, but to all those who value the good
health and abundant energy that good nutrition can
provide. The experiments cited above on newly weaned
infants show that humans as well as animals possess the
innate ability to select the foods that will provide the
optimal satisfaction of their nutritional needs of the hour.
The very young child has not yet acquired the prejudices
and taboos which are often generated by whatever
nutritional advice happens to be in vogue at the time.
Their taste discrimination is thus as keen as those of
animals in the wild. But, as Professor Richter says, 'Most
children are brought up by their parents to distrust their
own appetites. Often when they like a food, they are told

not to eat it, and when they dislike it they are equally often told that it is nourishing and good for them. In later life, such persons are much more apt to depend on food faddists than on their own taste sensations.'

References

Chapter 2

'Caution: very low-calorie diets can be deadly' in *Annals of Internal Medicine,* Editorial, vol. 102, p.121, 1985

Eyton, A., *The F-Plan,* Penguin, London, 1982

FDA Talk Paper: Cambridge Diet Update, US Department of Health, Education and Welfare publication (FDA) T82–95, Government Printing Office, 1982

Goette, D.K. and Odom, R.H., 'Profuse hair loss' in *Archives of Dermatology,* vol. 111, p.930, 1975

Herbert, V., *Nutrition Cultism, Facts and Fictions,* George F. Stickley Co., Philadelphia, 1980

– 'Will questionable nutrition overwhelm nutrition science?' in *American Journal of Clinical Nutrition,* vol. 34, p.2848, 1981

Howard, A., *The Cambridge Diet,* Cape, London, 1985

Isner, J.M., Sours, H.E., and Paris, A.L. *et al.,* 'Sudden unexpected deaths in avid dieters using the liquid protein modified fast diet' in *Circulation,* vol. 60, p.1401, 1979

Mazell, J., *The Beverly Hills Diet,* Macmillan Publishing Co Inc, New York, 1981

Mirkin, G.B. and Shore, R.N., 'The Beverly Hills Diet: dangers of the newest weight loss fad' in *Journal of the American Medical Association,* vol. 246, p.2235, 1981

Pritikin, N., *The Pritikin Permanent Weight Loss Manual,* Putnam Publishing Group, New York, 1981

Tarnowers, H. and Baker, S., *The Complete Scarsdale Medical Diet,* Bantam, London, 1980

Sours, H.E. *et al.*, 'Sudden death associated with very low calorie weight reduction regimens' in *American Journal of Clinical Nutrition*, vol. 34, p.453, 1981

Van Itallie, T.B., 'The liquid protein mayhem' in *Journal of the American Medical Association*, vol. 240, p.140, 1978

Wadden, T.A., Stunkard, A.J., Brownell, K.D. and Van Itallie, T.B., 'The Cambridge Diet: more mayhem?' in *Journal of the American Medical Association*, vol. 250, p.2833, 1983

Wilson, J.H.P. and Lamberts, S.W.J., 'Nitrogen balance in obese patients receiving a very low-calorie liquid formula diet' in *American Journal of Clinical Nutrition*, vol. 32, p.1612, 1979

Chapter 3

Himms-Hagen, J., 'Obesity may be due to a malfunctioning of brown fat' in *Canadian Medical Association Journal*, vol. 121, p. 1361, 1979

– 'Thyroid hormones and thermogenesis' in *Mammalian Thermogenesis*, Eds. Girardier, L. and Stock, N.J., Chapman and Hall, London, 1983

Jung, R.T., Shetty, O.S., James, W.P.T. *et al.*, 'Reduced thermogenesis in obesity' in *Nature*, vol. 279, p.323, 1979

Lewin, R., 'Overblown reports distort obesity risks' in *Science*, vol. 211, p. 258, 1981

McCloy, J. and McCloy, R.F., 'Encephalins, hunger and obesity' in *Lancet*, vol. 3, p. 753, 1979

Rothwell, N.J. and Stock, N.J., 'A role for brown adipose tissue in diet-induced thermogenesis' in *Nature*, vol. 281, p. 31, 1979

– 'Effect of chronic food restriction on energy balance,

thermogenic capacity, and brown-adipose tissue activity in the rat' in *Bioscience Reports*, vol. 2, p. 543, 1982

Schutz, Y. *et al.*, 'Diet-induced thermogenesis measured over a whole day in obese and non-obese women' in *American Journal of Clinical Nutrition*, vol. 40, p. 542, 1984

Shetty, P.S. *et al.*, 'Postprandial thermogenesis in obestiy' in *Clinical Science*, vol. 60, p. 519, 1961

Shimomura, Y. *et al.*, 'Opiate receptors, food intake and obesity' in *Physiology and Behavioiur*, vol. 28, p. 441, 1982

Chapter 4

Burkitt, D.P. and Trowell, H.C., *Refined carbohydrate foods and disease: the implications of dietary fibre*, Academic Press, London, 1975

Cohen, B., 'Scientific basis for the prevention of caries and periodontal disease' in *Proceedings of the Royal Society of Medicine*, vol. 74, p. 262, 1979

Darby, W.J., 'Some obsevations concerning nutrition and dental health' in *Journal of Clinical Periodontology*, vol. 6, p. 37, 1979

Diet and coronary heart disease, Committee on Medical Aspects of Food Policy (COMA) report, Department of Health and Social Security, London, 1984

'Does control of risk factors prevent coronary heart disease?', Editorial, *British Medical Journal,* vol. 2, pp.1065 and 1738, 1982

Gerutti, G. *et al.*, 'Phytic acid in bran and in "natural" foods' in *Bolletino Chimico Farmaceutico*, Milan

Kelsey, J.L., 'A review of research on effects of fiber intake on man' in *American Journal of Clinical Nutrition,* vol. 31, p.142, 1978

Keys, A., 'Atherosclerosis: a problem in newer public

health' in *Journal of the Mount Sinai Hospital,* vol. 20, p.118, 1953

– 'Prevention of coronary heart disease' in *Circulation,* vol. 38, p.227, 1968

Laragh, J.P. and Pecker, M.S., 'Dietary sodium and essential hypertension: some myths, hopes and truths' in *Annals of Internal Medicine,* vol. 98 (part 2), p. 735, 1983

Levitt, M.D. and Engel, R.R. 'intestinal gas' in *Advances in Internal Medicine,* vol. 20, p.151, 1975

Mann, G.V., 'Diet-heart: end of an era' in *New England Journal of Medicine,* vol. 297, p.644, 1977

McMichael, J., 'Dietary prevention of ischaemic heart disease' in *British Medical Journal,* vol. 2, p.1065, 1980

– 'Fats and atheroma: an inquest' in *British Medical Journal,* vol. 1, p.890, 1979

Mitchell, J.R.A., 'But will it help *my* patients with myocardial infarction? The implications of recent trials for everyday country folk' in *British Medical Journal,* vol. 2, p.1140, 1982

NACNE, *A discussion paper on proposals for nutritional guidelines for health education in Britain,* Health Education Council, London, 1983

Rao, D.C. *et al.* (Eds.), *Genetic epidemiology of coronary heart disease: past, present and future,* Alan R. Liss, New York, 1984

Roberts, I.F. *et al.,* 'Malnutrition in infants receiving cult diets' in *British Medical Journal,* vol. 1, p.296, 1979

Smith, J., 'Nutrition and the media' in *Preventive Nutrition and Society* (Ed. Turner, M.R.), Academic Press, London, 1981

Trowell, H., 'Indigestible residue or dietary fiber' in *American Journal of Clinical Nutrition,* vol. 36, p.194, 1982

– *Towards Healthful Diets*, National Academy of Sciences, Washington, 1980

Chapter 5

Chalmer, J., *et al.*, 'Anorexia nervosa presenting as morbid exercising' in *Lancet*, vol. 1, p.286, 1985

Cumming, D.C. *et al.*, 'Exercise and reproductive function in women' in *Progress in Clinical Biological Research*, vol. 117, p.113, 1983

Fonda, J., *Jane Fonda's Workout Book*, Penguin, London, 1984

Leblang, J., *et al.*, 'Effect of diet and exercise on norepinephrine-induced thermogenesis in male and female rats' in *Applied Physiology*, vol. 52, p.556, 1982

Chapter 6

Cabanac, M., 'Physiological role of pleasure' in *Science*, vol. 173, p.1103, 1971

Ciofti, L.A., James, W.P.T. and Van Itallie, T.B., *The body weight regulatory system: normal and disturbed mechanisms*, Raven Press, New York, 1981

Himms-Hagen, J., 'Thermogenesis in brown adipose tissue as an energy buffer: implications for obesity' in *New England Journal of Medicine*, vol. 311, p.1549, 1984

Perkins, M.N., Rothwell, N.J., Stock, N.J. and Stone, T.W., 'Activation of brown adipose tissue thermogenesis by the ventromedial hypothalamus' in *Nature*, vol. 289, p. 401, 1981

Rothwell, N.J. and Stock, N.J., 'Regulation of energy balance' in *Annual Review of Nutrition*, vol. 1, p. 235, 1981

– 'Diet-induced thermogenesis and brown fat: the case in favour' in *Clinical Science,* vol. 64, p.19, 1983

Shetty, P.S. *et al.,* 'Postprandial thermogenesis in obesity' in *Clinical Science,* vol. 60, p.519, 1981

Chapter 9

Arora, R.B. (Ed.), *Development of Unani drugs from herbal sources and the role of elements in their mechanism of action,* Hamdard National Foundation Monograph, Hamdard National Foundation, New Delhi, India, 1985

Appendix

Davis, C., 'Self-selection of diet by newly weaned infants' in *American Journal of Diseases of Children,* vol. 36, p.651, 1928

Himms-Hagen, J., Triandafillou, J. and Gwilliam, C., 'Brown adipose tissue of cafeteria-fed rats' in *American Journal of Physiology,* vol. 241, p. 116, 1981

Richter, C.P., 'Total self-regulatory functions in animals and human beings', *The Harvey Lectures,* series XXXVIII, 1943

Rothwell, J. *et al.,* 'Effect of feeding a "cafeteria" diet on energy balance and diet-induced thermogenesis in four strains of rat' in *Journal of Nutrition,* vol. 112, p.1515, 1982

Tepper, B.J. and Kanarek, R.B., 'Dietary self-selection patterns of rats with mild diabetes' in *Journal of Nutrition,* vol. 115, p.699, 1985

Index

Health and self-help books now available in Panther Books

W H Bates
Better Eyesight Without Glasses   £1.95 ☐

Ronald Gatty
The Body Clock Diet   £1.50 ☐

Desmonde Dunne
Yoga Made Easy   £1.95 ☐

Laurence E Morehouse & Leonard Gross
Total Fitness   £1.95 ☐
Maximum Performance   £1.50 ☐

Constance Mellor
Guide to Natural Health   £1.25 ☐
Natural Remedies for Common Ailments   £1.95 ☐

Sonya Richmond
Yoga and Your Health   £1.25 ☐

Phyllis Speight
Homoeopathy   £1.50 ☐

Kenneth Lysons
How to Cope with Hearing Loss   95p ☐

Dr Richard B Stuart
Act Thin, Stay Thin   £1.50 ☐

Dr Carl C Pfeiffer & Jane Banks
Total Nutrition   £1.50 ☐

Dr Hamilton Hall
Be Your Own Back Doctor   £1.95 ☐

José Silva and Michael Miele
The Silva Mind Control Method   £2.50 ☐

Dr Peter M Miller
The Change Your Metabolism Diet   £1.95 ☐

Slimming Magazine
30-Day Formula   £3.95 ☐

To order direct from the publisher just tick the titles you want and fill in the order form.   **HB881**

All these books are available at your local bookshop or newsagent, or can be ordered direct from the publisher.

To order direct from the publisher just tick the titles you want and fill in the form below.

Name _____

Address _____

Send to:
Panther Cash Sales
PO Box 11, Falmouth, Cornwall TR10 9EN.

Please enclose remittance to the value of the cover price plus:

UK 45p for the first book, 20p for the second book plus 14p per copy for each additional book ordered to a maximum charge of £1.63.

BFPO and Eire 45p for the first book, 20p for the second book plus 14p per copy for the next 7 books, thereafter 8p per book.

Overseas 75p for the first book and 21p for each additional book.

Panther Books reserve the right to show new retail prices on covers, which may differ from those previously advertised in the text or elsewhere.